Fatma ELLOUMI
Jamel DAOUD

Thymic epithelial tumors

Fatma ELLOUMI
Jamel DAOUD

Thymic epithelial tumors

Diagnosis and therapeutic management

ScienciaScripts

Imprint

Any brand names and product names mentioned in this book are subject to trademark, brand or patent protection and are trademarks or registered trademarks of their respective holders. The use of brand names, product names, common names, trade names, product descriptions etc. even without a particular marking in this work is in no way to be construed to mean that such names may be regarded as unrestricted in respect of trademark and brand protection legislation and could thus be used by anyone.

Cover image: www.ingimage.com

This book is a translation from the original published under ISBN 978-620-3-42446-1.

Publisher:
Sciencia Scripts
is a trademark of
Dodo Books Indian Ocean Ltd. and OmniScriptum S.R.L publishing group

120 High Road, East Finchley, London, N2 9ED, United Kingdom
Str. Armeneasca 28/1, office 1, Chisinau MD-2012, Republic of Moldova, Europe
Managing Directors: Ieva Konstantinova, Victoria Ursu
info@omniscriptum.com

Printed at: see last page
ISBN: 978-620-4-04087-5

Copyright © Fatma ELLOUMI, Jamel DAOUD
Copyright © 2021 Dodo Books Indian Ocean Ltd. and OmniScriptum S.R.L publishing group

Table of contents

- Table of contents 1
- Epidemiology of thymic epithelial tumors 3
  - Summary 3
  - I/Introduction 3
  - II/Frequency-Incidence 3
  - III/Age-Sex 4
  - IV /Etiopathogenesis/Facilitating factors 4
- Pathological aspects of thymic epithelial tumours 7
  - 1   Introduction 7
  - 2   Thymomas 8
  - 3   Thymic carcinoma 25
  - 4   Thymic neuroendocrine tumors 29
  - Annex 32
- Thymic epithelial tumors: clinical aspects and positive diagnosis 35
  - Summary 35
  - 1. Introduction 35
  - 2. Clinical signs 35
  - 3. Paraneoplastic syndromes 36
  - 4. Positive diagnosis 37
  - References 38
- Radiological aspects of thymic epithelial tumors 40
  - Summary 40
  - I- Introduction 40
  - II- The thoracic radiography 40
  - III- Contribution of thoracic computed tomography (CT) 41
  - References 44
- Minimally invasive surgery for thymoma: indications and approach 45
  - Summary 45
  - I- Introduction 45
  - II- Minimally invasive approaches for thymoma surgery 45
  - III- Surgical variants of minimally invasive approaches 48
  - IV- Indications for minimally invasive surgery 49
  - V- Results of minimally invasive surgery 52
  - References 56
- Surgery for locally invasive thymomas 59
  - Summary 59
  - I- Definition 59
  - References 68

Place of Radiotherapy in the Treatment of Thymus Epithelial Tumors 71
    Summary 71
    I-   Introduction 71
    II-   Post-operative radiotherapy 72
    III- Neoadjuvant radiotherapy 74
    IV- Exclusive radiotherapy 74
    V- Palliative radiotherapy 76
    VI-   Conclusion 77
    References 77
Radiotherapy of TETs: Technical aspects and side effects 82
    I-   Introduction 82
    II-   Contouring of target volumes 82
    III . Dose of radiation therapy 83
    IV. Risk-bearing organs (RBOs) and dose constraints 84
    V. Radiotherapy Techniques 85
Systemic treatment of thymic epithelial tumors 94
    Summary 94
    I.   Introduction 94
    II.   Chemotherapy 94
    III.   Targeted therapies 100
    IV- Immunotherapy 102
    V-   Conclusion 103
    References 103

Epidemiology of thymic epithelial tumors

Manel Mellouli[1,3], Fatma Elloumi[2,3]
(1) Laboratory of anatomy and pathological cytology, CHU Habib Bourguiba, Sfax
(2) Department of carcinological radiotherapy, CHU Habib Bourguiba, Sfax
(3) Faculty of Medicine, Sfax-Tunisia

Summary:

Thymic epithelial tumours include thymomas, thymic carcinomas and neuroendocrine neoplasia. These tumours are rare and represent about 20% of mediastinal tumours and about 50% of tumours of the anterior mediastinum. The average age at diagnosis of thymic epithelial tumors is between 50 and 60 years, but these tumors can be seen at any age. No factors favouring the development of thymic epithelial tumours have been identified to date.

I/Introduction:

Thymic epithelial tumours include thymomas (5 main subtypes: A, AB, B1, B2, and B3), thymic carcinomas and neuroendocrine neoplasia. They are derived, by definition, from the epithelial cell contingent of the thymus and are therefore mostly located in the middle tier of the anterior mediastinum. The relative frequency of ectopic thymic islets explains the possibility of TETs of different cervicomediastinal topographies in less than 10% of cases [1]. These tumors represent about 20% of mediastinal tumors and about 50% of anterior mediastinal tumors. The histopathological classification recommended today to classify and manage them is WHO 2021 [2]. However, it is recognized that using this classification, about 15-20% of tumors are of difficult classification even among experts.

II/Frequency-Incidence:

Thymic epithelial tumors (TET) are rare with an incidence of 0.13 to 0.32 per

100,000 person-years [3,4,5]. Their incidence is estimated at 250 new cases per year in France. Type A thymoma is one of the rarest subtypes of thymoma. In a review of more than 2400 thymomas reported in several international studies, type A thymoma accounts for 11.5% (3.1-26.2%) of all thymomas [2,5]. Type AB thymoma is one of the most common subtypes of thymoma and accounts for 25% of thymomas in most studies [2,4,5]. In the International Thymic Malignancy Interest Group (ITMIG) cohort and an independent meta-analysis, type A, AB thymoma accounted for 17%, 26%, 16% of thymomas respectively (Table 1) [2,4].

Table I: epidemiological characteristics of thymoma [2].

Type	Relative frequency (interval)	Age groups (years) (average)	Male to female ratio
Type A	11,5% (3,1%-26,2%)	8-88 (64)	1 :1,4
Type AB	25% (15%-43%)	11-89 (57)	1 :1,4
Type B1	17,5% (5,9%-52,8%)	4-83 (50)	1 :1,6
Type B2	26% (8%-41,1%)	4-83 (49)	1 :1
Type B3	16% (3,4%-35,1)	8-87 (55)	1 :0,8
Micronodular	1%	41-83 (65)	1,2 :1
Metaplastic	<1%	28-71 (50)	1 :1,5

III/Age-Sex:

The average age at diagnosis of TETs is between 50 and 60 years (mean age is 58 years) [1-3]. These tumors rarely affect children. There is no gender-related predisposition, although a trend toward a female preponderance has been reported for subtypes A, AB, and B1, and a male preponderance for carcinomas [2,6-10]

IV /Etiopathogenesis/Favouring factors:

No factors favouring the development of thymic epithelial tumours, particularly environmental or infectious, have been identified to date. Data reporting the occurrence of thymoma after exposure to ionizing radiation, in immunocompromised individuals, including the context of human immunodeficiency virus (HIV) infection, or after solid organ transplantation, are difficult to interpret, especially in the context of differential diagnosis with rebound thymic hyperplasia, which is common in these situations. Some genetic diseases, such as multiple endocrine neoplasia type 1 (MEN 1), are associated with a higher incidence of thymic tumors, thymomas and thymic carcinoids, in a familial context and association with cancer susceptibility syndromes [11]. In addition, patients with a history of thymic epithelial tumor have an increased risk of developing extra-thymic, hematopoietic (diffuse large B-cell lymphomas and leukemias), and solid cancers (gastric, colorectal, pancreatic, thyroid cancers) [12]; these associations could correspond as much to the existence of common etiological factors or to a deficit in the mechanisms of antitumor immunity, as to adverse effects of the treatments implemented or to monitoring biases.

References:

1. Riedel RF, Burfeind Jr WR. Thymoma: benign appearance, malignant potential. Oncologist 2006;11:887-94.
2. The WHO Classification of Tumours Editorial Board. WHO Classification of Thoracic Tumours. 5th Edition. Lyon: IARC Press; 2021: 320-398
3. Hsu CH, Chan JK, Yin CH, Lee CC, Chern CU, Liao CI. Trends in the incidence of thymoma, thymic carcinoma, and thymic neuroendocrine tumor in the United States. PLoS One. 2019 Dec 31;14(12):e0227197.
4. Weis CA, Yao X, Deng Y, Detterbeck FC, Marino M, Nicholson AG, Huang J, Ströbel P, Antonicelli A, Marx A; Contributors to the ITMIG Retrospective Database. The impact of thymoma histotype on prognosis in a worldwide database. J Thorac Oncol. 2015 Feb;10(2):367-72.
5. de Jong WK, Blaauwgeers JL, Schaapveld M, Timens W, Klinkenberg TJ, Groen HJ. Thymic epithelial tumours: a population-based study of the

incidence, diagnostic procedures and therapy. Eur J Cancer. 2008 Jan;44(1):123-30.
6. Marx A, Ströbel P, Badve SS, Chalabreysse L, Chan JK, Chen G, et al. ITMIG consensus statement on the use of the WHO histological classification of thymoma and thymic carcinoma: refined definitions, histological criteria, and reporting. J Thorac Oncol 2014;9:596-611.
7. Kondo K, Monden Y. Therapy for thymic epithelial tumors: a clinical study of 1,320 patients from Japan. Ann Thorac Surg 2003;76:878-84.
8. Weis CA, Yao X, Deng Y, Detterbeck FC, Marino M, Nicholson AG, et al. Contributors to the ITMIG Retrospective Database. The impact of thymoma histotype on prognosis in a worldwide database. J Thorac Oncol 2015;10:367-72.
9. Ruffini E, Detterbeck F, Van Raemdonck D, Rocco G, Thomas P, Weder W, et al; European Association of Thoracic Surgeons (ESTS) Thymic Working Group. Tumours of the thymus: a cohort study of prognostic factors from the European Society of Thoracic Surgeons database. Eur J Cardiothorac Surg 2014;46:361-8.
10. Omasa M, Date H, Sozu T, Sato T, Nagai K, Yokoi K, et al; for the Japanese Association for Research on the Thymus. Postoperative radiotherapy is effective for thymic carcinoma but not for thymoma in stage II and III thymic epithelial tumors: The Japanese Association for Research on the Thymus Database Study. Cancer 2015;121:1008-16.
11. Kojima Y, Ito H, Hasegawa S, Sasaki T, Inui K. Resected invasive thymoma with multiple endocrine neoplasia type 1. Jpn J Thorac Cardiovasc Surg 2006;54:171-3.
12. Engels EA, Pfeiffer RM. Malignant thymoma in the United States: demographic patterns in incidence and associations with subsequent malignancies. Int J Cancer 2003;105:546-551.

Pathological aspects of thymic epithelial tumors

Meriam Triki[1,2], Marwa Bouhamed[1,2], Slim Charfi[1,2]

(1) Laboratory of Anatomy and Cytology Pathology, CHU Habib Bourguiba, Sfax, Tunisia

(2) Faculty of Medicine, Sfax, Tunisia

Summary

Thymic epithelial tumors are rare tumors with variable progression and prognosis. Many classifications have been developed over the years. The reference histological classification is that of the WHO updated in 2021, which distinguishes 3 main entities: thymomas, thymic carcinomas and thymic neuroendocrine tumours. Each of these entities is distinguished by a morphological aspect and an immunohistochemical profile quite characteristic. The staging system most often used is that of Masaoka, revised by Koga.

1 Introduction:

Thymic tumours are the most common tumour of the anterior superior mediastinum. They represent 20% to 30% of all mediastinal tumours and about half of the masses of the anterior mediastinum (1). Thymus tumors constitute a complex entity integrating thymic epithelial tumors and other rarer lesions developing in the thymic cavity. Their morphological diversity and architectural complexity make their study difficult. Thymic epithelial tumors are rare (2). They include thymomas, thymic carcinomas and thymic neuroendocrine tumours (3).

2 Thymomas:

2.1 Definition:

Thymomas are defined by the presence of a dual lymphocytic reaction and epithelial tumor contingent. The epithelial contingent is responsible for the aggressiveness of the tumor, hence its consideration as a malignant tumor, even in the absence of microscopic invasion. This is justified by its potential for local invasion, recurrence or distant metastasis (3).

2.2 WHO pathology classification (Appendix I) :

The new edition of the WHO classification of thoracic tumours published in 2021 maintains the use of a letter (A, B) and number (1, 2, 3) system for the classification of thymic tumours. This system has been in use since the WHO edition published in 1999 (3).

Type A: A tumor composed of spindle cells without nuclear atypia accompanied by a negligible lymphocytic contingent.

Type AB: A tumor with type A areas similar to those described above and type B areas rich in lymphocytes.

Type B1: Organoid tumor resembling a functional thymus with predominantly dark areas of thymic cortex and minority light areas of thymic medulla.

Type B2: Tumor composed of thymic epithelial cells with abundant cytoplasm and vesicular and nucleolated nuclei, dispersed in an abundant non-tumorous immature lymphocyte population. Perivascular spaces are frequently encountered with a palisading arrangement of epithelial cells at their contact.

Type B3: Tumour composed essentially of round or polygonal epithelial cells with atypia at most moderate.

Besides these tumors, the WHO recognizes three other rarer histological types of thymoma:

Micronodular type with lymphoid stroma: tumor composed of epithelial cells separated by a lymphoid background.

Metaplastic type: biphasic tumor with epithelial and spindle cells.

Lipofibroadenoma: tumor resembling the fibroadenoma of the breast with a predominantly hyaline fibrous stroma, pushing back the epithelial cells, with the presence of adipocytes and some lymphocytes.

Note that microscopic and sclerosing types are no longer recognized as types of thymoma by the new WHO 2021 classification.

2.3 Thymoma A :

2.3.1 Macroscopy:

A well-limited, encapsulated tumour, homogeneous in appearance on section, whitish or brownish in colour, with an average size of 7.2 cm.

2.3.2 Microscopy:

It is a lobulated tumor, completely or incompletely encapsulated. This tumor is composed essentially of thymic epithelial cells spindle or oval (rarely polygonal), regular, with fine chromatin and a discrete nucleolus. The mitotic index is low, often less than 4 mitoses /2mm2. These cells are accompanied by a negligible or absent immature lymphocytic contingent. Occupation of more than 10% of the tumor surface by TDT+ lymphocytes reclassifies the tumor as AB thymoma.

Several architectural aspects have been described and may coexist in the same tumor: fasciculated, storiform, hemangiopericytic, rosettes with or without central lumen, glomeruloid, glandular, meningioma-like or hemangioma-like with pseudopapillary intra-cystic projection.

Perivascular spaces are less observed than in other types of thymomas with absence of Hassal's corpuscle.

The absence of Hassal's corpuscle, storiform architecture, pseudo-rosettes, clusters of foamy histiocytes and pseudo-glandular structures characterize this lesion.

A variant of atypical thymoma A was individualized by the 2015 WHO classification and is maintained in the 2021 WHO classification. It has the same histological features as type A thymoma but differs in the presence of atypia (hypercellularity, high mitotic index, focal necrosis).

2.3.3 Immunohistochemistry:

The epithelial cells express AE1, P63 and PAX8. They are negative for CK20 and AE3, CD5 and CD117. Focal CD20 labeling by epithelial cells can be observed (which may be negative on biopsy). EMA expression is variable and focal.

TDT may mark rare immature CD3+ T cells but is often negative. CD20+ B cells are usually absent.

2.3.4 Differential diagnosis:

The differential diagnosis is mainly with solitary fibrous tumors (CK-, STAT6+, CD34+) and synovial sarcoma

2.3.5 Prognosis:

The average age of survival at 5 and 10 years is close to 100%. After 5 to 10 years the recurrence rate is 5 to 10%.

2.4 **Thymoma AB** :

2.4.1 Macroscopy

This tumor is often encapsulated with a nodular appearance separated by whitish fibrous septa. The average size varies from 7 to 8 cm.

2.4.2 Microscopy

Histologically, the tumor is lobulated, well-bounded, often with lymphocyte-poor A-type foci and B-like foci characterized by the presence of clusters of immature TDT+ lymphocytes (difficult to count) (Figure 1A).

These two contingents may form separate lobules or be intertwined.

The architecture of the A contingent is variable and may take the form of spindle cell bundles surrounding lymphocyte-rich B-like nodules.

The B-like contingent consists of small oval or polygonal cells with round or oval, finely nucleated nuclei.

The presence of large nucleated vesicular nuclei characteristic of type B2 is rarely seen. Medullary islands are rare and Hassal's corpuscles are usually absent.

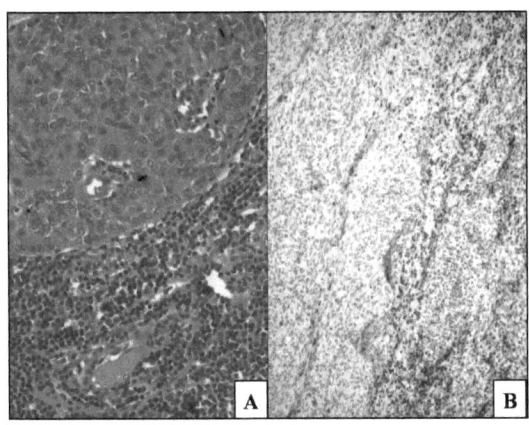

Figure 1: AB thymoma: **(A)** Presence of a lymphocyte-poor type A focus in contact with a lymphocyte-rich type B-like focus (HEx200). **(B)** Positive immunostaining for TDT in the lymphocytes of the B-like contingent (x100).

2.4.3 Immunohistochemistry:

Epithelial cells of the A and B contingent express pankeratin, P63/P40 and CD20. They are negative for CD5. Spindle cells are strongly positive for vimentin and EMA and weakly positive for pankeratin.

The lymphocytes are predominantly immature T cells (CD3 and TDT positive) (Figure 1B). CD20+ B cells are generally absent.

Ki 67 is low in epithelial cells but interpretation is difficult due to the large number of immature T cells.

2.4.4 Differential diagnosis:

The differential diagnosis is with thymoma A and micronodular thymoma.

Any thymoma with lymphocyte-poor type A foci associated with areas rich in TDT-positive immature T cells (cannot be counted) or foci showing a moderate infiltrate of TDT+ immature T cells (difficult to count) that is greater than 10% of the tumor area should be classified as AB thymoma.

Micronodular thymoma is distinguished by a lymphoid stroma rich in CD20-positive B cells and located outside the epithelial nodules.

2.4.5 Prognosis:

Overall survival is 80%-100% at 5 and 10 years. Recurrence and metastasis are rare. The recurrence rate at 10 years is 3-5% after surgical resection.

2.5 Thymoma B1 :

2.5.1 Macroscopy:

It is an often encapsulated or well-limited tumor ranging in size from 5.1 to 7.5 cm. On section, it is yellowish in colour with a nodular and lobulated appearance, separated by septa. Cystic and necrotic changes may be seen.

2.5.2 Microscopy

Histologically, the tumor architecture is organoid, resembling a functional thymus with predominantly dark and light areas. Epithelial cells are rare, scattered and not grouped in clusters. They are barely detectable at low magnification. An increase in cell density or the presence of clusters of more than 3 epithelial cells reclassifies the tumour as a B2 thymoma.

These cells have vesicular oval nuclei with a small central nucleolus and pale eosinophilic cytoplasm. They are intermingled with numerous TDT positive T cells. Spindle cells are absent. Their presence reclassifies the tumor as AB thymoma.

Pale, less cellular nodular areas with mature B and T cells corresponding to foci of marrow differentiation are mandatory for positive diagnosis; however, they are not specific and may be found in AB and B2 thymomas.

Large perivascular spaces and Hassal's corpuscles are often present. An association with a B2 thymoma occurs in 20% of cases and with a B3 thymoma is rarer.

2.5.3 Immunohistochemistry:

Epithelial cells express CK19, AE1/AE3, P63; they are negative for CK20 and CD20. Lymphocytes in the cortical area are marked by TdT, CD1a and CD3.

The medullary islets are characterized by mature T cells (CD3 positive, TdT and CD1a negative), and CD20 positive B cells.

2.5.4 Differential diagnosis:

The differential diagnosis arises with:

Normal thymus: this is formed by lobules surrounded by fat cells rather than fibrous septa. However, the distinction may be impossible on biopsy.

B2 thymoma: the epithelial cells are grouped in clusters (with a denser positive marking to cytokeratins), in addition the presence of medullary islands with or without Hassal's corpuscle is obligatory in type B1 whereas they are rare in type B2.

AB thymoma: it is distinguished by the presence of spindle cell foci.

The epithelial cells are more numerous and express cytokeratin and CD20.

T lymphoblastic lymphoma: this tumor usually occurs in children and adolescents. It leads to an effacement of the cortico-medullary architecture with infiltration of the mediastinal fat. The tumor cells are more monotonous, more atypical and slightly larger than a thymocyte. Several mitoses, apoptotic bodies or necrosis are observed.

To avoid misdiagnosis, it is recommended to request an epithelial marker panel including cytokeratins and P63.

2.5.5 Prognosis:

The overall survival rate is 80-100% at 5 and 10 years. Recurrence of TNM stage I tumors is seen in 10% of cases after 10 years of follow-up.

2.6 Thymoma B2 :

2.6.1 Macroscopy:

The tumor may be encapsulated or poorly limited with invasion of mediastinal fat or adjacent organs.

Its average diameter varies from 4 to 6.2 cm. On section, it is yellowish in colour, soft to firm in consistency, and lobulated by whitish fibrous septa. Hemorrhagic, necrotic and cystic changes may be seen (Figure 2).

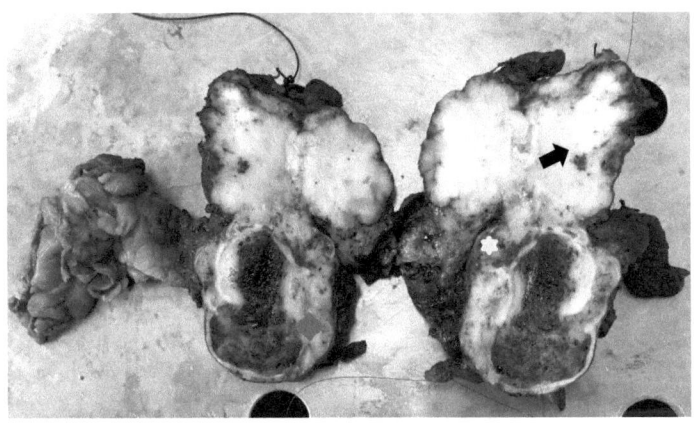

Figure 2: Macroscopic appearance of a B2 Thymoma: Yellowish tumor with poor fat infiltration ( )(Masaoka-Koga IIb stage) with hemorrhagic ( ) and necrotic ( ) changes

2.6.2 Microscopy:

Microscopically, the tumor appears blue due to its richness in lymphocytes.

It is arranged in lobules of irregular size and shape, separated by fibrous septa (Figure 3).

T cells are mixed with polygonal or oval epithelial cells, arranged singly or in small clusters (more than 3 cells). These cells have round or oval nuclei with a vesicular appearance and a small prominent nucleolus.

Rare cases may show an anaplastic appearance that remains focal. Perivascular spaces, characterized by a central venule surrounded by a clear space with a few lymphocytes, are frequently encountered.

Medullary spaces with or without Hassal's corpuscles are rare.

Lymphoid follicles may be present in the fibrous septa or in the perivascular spaces.

Association with a B3 or B1 thymoma can be seen in 43% and 4% of cases respectively. The association with a thymic carcinoma is exceptional.

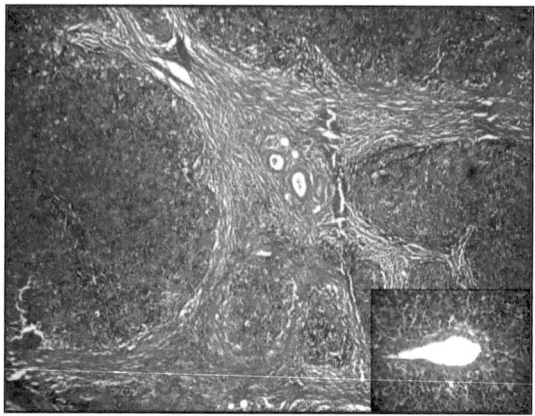

Figure 3: Thymoma B2: Tumour proliferation arranged in lobules of irregular size and shape, separated by fibrous septa (HEx100). **Inset**: Presence of perivascular space with surrounding palisading of epithelial cells (HEx200).

2.6.3 Immunohistochemistry:

The epithelial cells are positive for cytokeratins and P63/P40 (denser labelling than in thymoma B1), negative for CD20.

These cells are mixed with immature TDT-positive lymphocytes. CD20 positive B cells are present in the rare marrow spaces.

2.6.4 Differential diagnosis

It lands with :

Thymoma B1: In this tumor, epithelial cells are rare and are not grouped in clusters. The medullary spaces are always present and mandatory for the diagnosis. The perivascular spaces are less prominent.

Thymoma B3: This is a tumour with a low lymphocyte count. The presence of a diffuse patch of epithelial cells gives a pink coloration to the microscopic examination contrary to the B2 thymoma which has a blue color due to its richness in lymphocyte.

T lymphoblastic lymphoma can mimic a lymphocyte-rich thymoma (Type B1 and B2).

B2 thymoma with anaplasia can be distinguished from thymic carcinoma by the presence of the typical thymoma features of lobulated architecture, perivascular spaces, TDT positive immature T cells and absence of CD5/CD117 expression.

2.6.5 Prognosis:

Survival at 5 years is 70 to 100%. It is 45 to 82% at 10 years. Complete resection is obtained in 70 to 90% of cases. The recurrence rate after complete resection in TNM stage I tumours is 14% and 32% at 5 and 10 years respectively.

2.7 Thymoma B3 :

2.7.1 Macroscopy:

Macroscopically, the tumor is often poorly limited, with invasion of mediastinal fat and neighboring organs.

The average diameter varies from 5.1 cm to 6.8 cm.

On section, it has a yellowish-grey colouring, sometimes with haemorrhagic and necrotic changes.

2.7.2 Microscopy:

The tumor is formed by nodules of irregular size and shape delimited by fibrous septa.

At low magnification, the tumor appears pink due to the abundance of polygonal epithelial cells with clarified eosinophilic cytoplasm, arranged in diffuse patches (Figure 4).

Their nuclei show moderate atypia at most. They are round or irregular oval, sometimes incised, with a discrete or prominent nucleolus.

These epithelial cells take on a palisading arrangement around the prominent perivascular spaces.

Rare immature T cells are almost always present scattered within this proliferation. However, they may be absent in less than 5% of cases.

Rarely, spindle cells or foci of anaplasia characterized by giant or bizarre tumor cells may be seen.

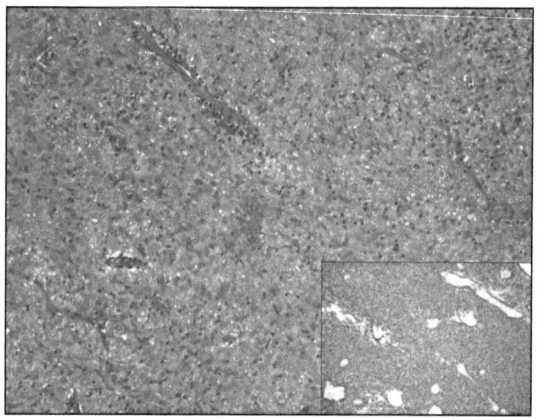

Figure 4: Thymoma B3: Tumor proliferation made of epithelial-like cells, diffusely arranged in a palisading perivascular pattern, with the presence of rare scattered lymphocytes (HEx200). **Inset**: Positive immunostaining for cytokeratin (x200).

2.7.3 Immunohistochemistry:

Epithelial tumor cells express cytokeratin (Figure 4), P63, P40, CK19, CK5/6 and CK7. They are negative for CK20.

CD20, TTF1 and thymic carcinoma markers (CD5 and CD117) are almost always negative or focal.

TdT marks rare immature T cells in over 95% of cases.

2.7.4 Differential diagnosis:

It occurs with Thymoma B2 and squamous cell carcinoma.

Squamous cell carcinoma can be distinguished from B3 thymoma by the absence of lobulated architecture and perivascular spaces. The atypia is more severe. On immunohistochemistry, CD5 (75% of cases) and CD117 (>80% of cases) positivity is noted with absence of immature TdT positive lymphocytes.

2.7.5 Prognosis:

The overall survival is 60-86%, 50-70%, 25-36% at 5, 10 and 20 years respectively. The complete removal rate varies from 53% to 92%. Recurrence is seen in 23% and 29% of all stages at 5 and 10 years respectively.

2.8 Micronodular thymoma with lymphoid stroma :

2.8.1 Macroscopy:

It is a well-limited tumour, often encapsulated, with a soft or friable consistency, homogeneous in appearance on section, with occasional cystic remodelling. The diameter varies from 1.2 to 15 cm

2.8.2 Microscopy:

It is characterized by the presence of multiple small, discrete and/or coalescing epithelial nodules separated by abundant lymphoid stroma, often containing lymphoid follicles with or without germinal centers and numerous plasma cells. The epithelial cells are small, oval or spindle-shaped, regular, with sparse cytoplasm and an oval or elongated, finely nucleated nucleus. They sometimes form pseudo-rosettes or glandular formations. Micro and macro cystic changes are frequent. Hassal's corpuscles and perivascular spaces are absent.

Association with Thymoma A is seen in 30% of cases. It is rarer with AB, B2 thymoma and thymic carcinoma.

2.8.3 Immunohistochemistry:

The epithelial cells are positive for pankeratin, CK5/6, CK19 and negative for CD20. Within these nodules, rare immature T lymphocytes (TdT positive) are present

Within the lymphoid stroma, pankeratin immunostaining is negative (no epithelial cells). There are mostly mature B cells (CD20 positive) mixed with some mature (CD3 positive, TdT negative) and immature (CD3, TdT, CD1a and CD99 positive) T cells.

2.8.4 Differential diagnosis:

It lands with :

Thymic follicular hyperplasia: In this case, Hassal's corpuscles and lobulated thymic architecture are maintained.

AB thymoma: In this case, the lymphocyte-rich areas contain pankeratin-positive epithelial cells. Lymphocytes are mostly immature (TdT positive) but B lymphocytes are rare.

Micronodular carcinoma with lymphoid hyperplasia: It is distinguished by the presence of frank atypia and by the absence of immature T cells in the lymphoid stroma.

2.8.5 Prognosis:

The majority of cases are Masaoka stage I/II. Recurrence, metastasis or death after surgical resection have never been reported.

2.9 Metaplastic thymoma:

2.9.1 Macroscopy:

It presents as an often well-limited, encapsulated mass, rarely with invasive borders. It is greyish-white or yellowish in appearance, and fasciculated on section. The average size varies from 3 to 18 cm.

2.9.2 Microscopy:

It is a biphasic thymoma with two contingents: epithelial and spindle cell, of variable proportion and essential for positive diagnosis. The transition between these two contingents may be abrupt or progressive. There is no lobular architecture or perivascular spaces.

The epithelial component is made up of islands or cords of oval or polygonal cells, showing in some places squamous differentiation or images of cell windings. These cells have vesicular incised nuclei, sometimes nucleolated, or may be large, pleomorphic with intranuclear inclusions. Mitosis figures are rare.

The spindle cell component is fasciculated or storiform in architecture, with regular cells that are rarely atypical. There are often a few lymphocytes and plasma cells scattered within this proliferation. Areas of focal necrosis have been reported rarely.

Rare cases of sarcomatoid carcinoma have been described in association with metaplastic thymoma suggesting transformation to a high grade tumor.

2.9.3 Immunohistochemistry:

Epithelial cells are positive for pankeratin, p63, p40, EMA (variable) and negative for vimentin.

Spindle cells mark vimentin diffusely and smooth muscle actin, EMA and pankeratin weakly. They are negative for p63 and p40.

Both contingents are negative for CD5, CD20, CD34 and CD117 with a low Ki67 (<5%)

Immature T cells are absent. Anti-TdT antibody is negative but may be positive in a residual thymic focus.

2.9.4 Differential diagnosis:

It lands with :

Sarcomatoid carcinoma (carcinosarcoma): this tumor shows a high grade fusocellular component with obvious atypia, numerous mitoses, necrosis with sometimes an associated heterologous component.

Thymoma A: seen in the absence of immature T cells and the presence of a variable epithelial contingent. However, it is typically a monophasic tumor that lacks anastomosing islands of polygonal cells with a squamous appearance. In addition, the spindle cells strongly and diffusely express pankeratin and CD20 while being negative for vimentin.

2.9.5 Prognosis:

The median overall survival after surgical excision reported in the literature was 10 years. One patient developed a recurrence at 14 months and died after 6 years. Two patients had transformation to sarcomatoid carcinoma at the time of diagnosis.

2.10 Thymus lipofibroadenoma:

2.10.1 Macroscopy:

It is an oval, well-limited tumor with a diameter ranging from 3 to 23 cm. On section, it has a firm solid consistency with a greyish colour.

2.10.2 Microscopy:

This tumor resembles the fibroadenoma of the breast with a predominantly hyaline fibrous stroma, displacing the monotonous epithelial cells arranged in trabeculae. There are associated adipocytes and some lymphocytes. Hassal's corpuscles and calcifications may be seen. Three cases were associated with an adjacent B1 thymoma.

2.10.3 Immunohistochemistry:

Epithelial cells label AE1/AE3 and CK19. Lymphocytes are polymorphic expressing CD3 and CD20 with absence of TdT labelling.

2.10.4 Differential diagnosis:

It lands with :

Thymolipoma: this is a predominantly adipose tumour with no fibrous contingent.

Thymofibrolipoma: is a subtype of thymolipoma, with a predominantly fibrous component.

It is currently unclear whether the entities thymolipoma, thymofibrolipoma and lipofibroadenoma belong to the same neoplastic or hamartomatous spectrum.

Sclerosing thymoma: this tumor is characterized by a dense collagenous background surrounding large islands of polygonal epithelial cells with absence of adipocytes.

2.10.5 Prognosis:

It is a benign tumor (no recurrence reported in the literature after complete resection).

2.11 Masaoka classification (Appendix II) :

Masaoka's clinical classification is the most commonly used to classify thymomas.

I: Completely encapsulated tumor without capsule invasion.

IIa: Microscopic invasion of the capsule.

IIb: Macroscopic invasion of the capsule and/or mediastinal fat.

III: Microscopic or macroscopic invasion of neighbouring organs (pleura, pericardium, lung, large mediastinal vessels, nerves).

IVa: Pleural or pericardial metastases.

IVb: distant metastases.

3 Thymic carcinoma:

3.1 Definition:

Thymic carcinomas are rare mediastinal malignancies that are difficult to diagnose and manage. These tumors are classified as thymic epithelial tumors according to the WHO 2021 classification (3).

3.2 Macroscopy:

Macroscopically, thymic carcinomas present as non-encapsulated, greyish-white tumours with cystic, haemorrhagic and/or necrotic changes.

3.3 Microscopy:

The diagnosis of thymic carcinoma is a diagnosis of exclusion. It is based on the absence of the attributes of thymoma which are lobulated architecture and the coexistence of an epithelial component and an immature lymphocytic contingent. In addition, thymic metastasis should be ruled out. These tumors have no morphological features and are similar in all respects to tumors that may be found elsewhere than in the thymus. The RYTHMIC Network in its 2012 update of thymic epithelial tumors established diagnostic criteria for thymic carcinomas:

Diagnostic criteria for thymic carcinomas

Major criteria (necessary)
- Epithelial cell atypia
- Exclusion of the diagnosis of thymoma with atypia or anaplasia

• Exclusion of thymic metastasis, germ cell or epithelioid mesenchymal tumor

Minor (typical) criteria

• Infiltrating architecture

• Absence of immature TdT (+) lymphocytes

• Expression by epithelial cells of CD5, CD117(KIT), GLUT1 and MUC1.

3.3.1 Thymic squamous cell carcinoma:

It is arranged in trabeculae, islets and cords (Figure 5A), surrounded by a sclerohyaline stroma. In contrast to nonthymic squamous cell carcinomas, these tumors have rounded, minimally infiltrative outlines. The tumor cells are jointed, medium to large in size, with fairly abundant cytoplasm and atypical, vesicular or hyperchromatic nuclei. Keratinization may be observed in some cases, simulating Hassal's corpuscles. These tumors show variable differentiation depending on the presence of keratinization, the degree of nuclear pleomorphism and the extent of keratinizing maturation.

Micronodular carcinoma with lymphoid hyperplasia is a subtype of thymic squamous cell carcinoma with a marked similarity to micronodular thymoma.

In immunohistochemistry, the tumor cells express p63/p40 (Figure 5B) and PAX 8 (75%). They also express CD5 (Figure 5C), CD117, GLUT1 and MUC 1 (80%). These markers, although they may be focally expressed by thymomas, seem to be quite specific to thymic carcinomas.

Differential diagnoses are represented by thymic metastases of squamous cell carcinoma, thymoma type B3 and other types of thymic carcinoma (lymphoepithelial carcinoma, basaloid carcinoma, NUT carcinoma, sarcomatoid carcinoma), atypical carcinoid tumor or large cell neuroendocrine carcinoma. In these cases, morphology and immunohistochemical data play an important role.

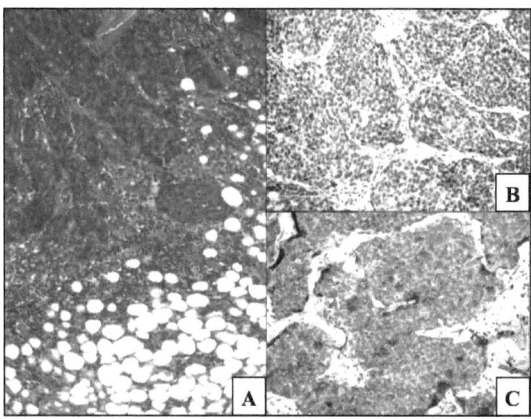

Figure 5: Poorly differentiated thymic squamous cell carcinoma: **(A)** Presence of carcinomatous proliferation arranged in clusters infiltrating the mediastinal fat (HEx100).
(B) Positive immunostaining for P63 (x100). **(C)** Membrane positive immunostaining for CD5 (x200).

3.3.2 Basaloid carcinoma :

The tumor cells are arranged in papillary, cystic, and nest-like structures. The cystic structures are lined by small cells in a palisading arrangement with rare papillary protrusions. The tumor cells are round or vaguely spindle-shaped, with unclear cytoplasmic boundaries. They have large, atypical, hyperchromatic, nucleated nuclei. The mitotic index may exceed 30 mitoses/ 2 mm2. Squamous differentiation is observed in 40% of cases.

On immunohistochemistry, the tumor cells express p63, p40 and CD117.

They express CD5 in less than 50% of cases.

The main differential diagnoses are thymic carcinoma with adenoid-cystic like aspects, large cell neuroendocrine carcinoma, NUT carcinoma and poorly differentiated squamous cell carcinoma. The palisading arrangement of the cells as well as their immunohistochemical profile represent real diagnostic keys.

3.3.3 Lymphoepithelial carcinoma:

Microscopically, these tumors are similar in every way to nasopharyngeal carcinomas. Indeed, the tumor cells present a cohesive aspect and are provided with large vesicular nuclei. Foci of fusocellular or squamous differentiation are described. Tumor cells often express PDL1, suggesting a key role of Epstein Bar Virus infection in their pathogenesis. On immunohistochemistry, tumor cells express pankeratin, p63, p40 and CD117. CD5 positivity is variable.

The main differential diagnoses are undifferentiated carcinoma (EBV negative), squamous cell carcinoma and metastasis of lymphoepithelial carcinoma from other locations. The cohesive appearance of the cells and their immunohistochemical profile are key elements in the diagnosis.

3.3.4 NUT carcinoma of the thorax:

It is a poorly differentiated carcinoma characterized by a rearrangement of the NUT gene.

The tumor cells are organized in nests and patches. They are monomorphic, small to medium in size, with irregular, vesicular nuclei and a prominent nucleolus. Rare foci of keratinization are observed (33%). An inflammatory infiltrate rich in neutrophils is often associated.

On immunohistochemistry, tumor cells express the NUT protein. They also express cytokeratin, p63, p40 and occasionally chromogranin, synaptophysin or TTF1.

The differential diagnosis is with poorly differentiated squamous cell carcinoma, small cell carcinoma, undifferentiated carcinoma and the spectrum of blue round cell tumours (Ewing's sarcoma and lymphomas).

3.3.5 Other Carcinomas :

- Clear cell carcinoma
- Low grade papillary adenocarcinoma
- Mucoepidermoid carcinoma
- Thymic carcinoma with cystic adenoid-like aspects
- Enteric-type adenocarcinoma
- NOS adenocarcinoma
- Adenosquamous carcinoma
- Sarcomatoid carcinoma
- Undifferentiated carcinoma
- Thymic carcinoma of the NOS type
-

4 Thymic neuroendocrine tumors:
4.1 Definition:

Pulmonary and thymic neuroendocrine tumors constitute a distinct class of tumors with morphological and biological neuroendocrine properties. They are classified into 4 histological types corresponding to 3 classes of increasing malignancy:

typical low-grade carcinoids,

Atypical carcinoids of intermediate grade,

-large cell neuroendocrine carcinoma (LCNEC) and high-grade small cell carcinoma.

They range from well-differentiated carcinoid neuroendocrine carcinomas to poorly differentiated small cell neuroendocrine carcinomas.

4.2 Macroscopy:

These tumours are non-encapsulated, large, with a firm but not lobulated, whitish-grey cross-section. Necrotic and hemorrhagic changes are present in 70% of cases and calcifications in 30%.

4.3 Microscopy:

Carcinoid tumors: The vast majority of thymic carcinoids are atypical carcinoids. They have in common that they often present with a more diffuse architecture, more marked cytonuclear atypia, and present at more advanced stages. The stroma is particularly desmoplastic, richly vascularized, often with invasion of lymphatic and blood vessels. Calcifications are noted in 30% of cases. The tumor cells have a granular cytoplasm and an atypical nucleus with slightly coarse chromatin.

Depending on the number of mitoses, and the presence of necrosis, these tumors will be classified into typical and atypical carcinoids with different prognosis. Atypical carcinoids are characterized by the presence of focal necrosis and/or a mitotic index of 2 to 10 mitoses /2mm2 (Appendix III).

On immunohistochemistry, tumor cells express Cytokeratin, EMA, NSE, Chromogranin, Synaptophysin and NCAM (CD56).

Special attention to the atypical carcinoid tumor with high mitotic index: similar to the grade 3 neuroendocrine tumor of the pancreas, it presents a morphology of carcinoid tumor but with a mitotic index > 10 / 2mm2. These tumors are still classified as NECC, but in the report, it should be specified that the histological appearance is that of a carcinoid tumor. The therapeutic approach is not the same as that of NSCLC.

Large cell neuroendocrine carcinoma (LCNEC) and thymic small cell carcinoma (TCC): They do not present any histological particularity differentiating them from their pulmonary counterparts. The main difficulty is to distinguish them from thymic metastases of carcinomas of pulmonary origin. They are also capable of presenting a non-neuroendocrine contingent and are then termed composite NSCLC or composite CPC.

References:
1. Dautzenberg B. Thymus tumors. Pneumology [Internet]. 1995; Available from: http://www.sciencedirect.com/science/article/pii/s1155195x95069983

2. de Jong WK, Blaauwgeers JL, Schaapveld M, Timens W, Klinkenberg TJ, Groen HJ. Thymic epithelial tumours: a population-based study of the incidence, diagnostic procedures and therapy. Eur J Cancer. 2008;44(1):123-30.

3. Chan J, Lantuejoul S, Marks A. Tumours of the Thymus. In: World Health Organization Classification of Tumours 5th edition Thoracic Tumours. Lyon: IARC press. 2021. p. 319-97.

4. Detterbeck FC, Nicholson AG, Kondo K, Van Schil P, Moran C. The Masaoka-Koga stage classification for thymic malignancies: clarification and definition of terms. J ThoracOncol. 2011;6(7):S1710-6.

Appendix I: Classification of thymic tumours according to the WHO classification of thoracic tumours published in 2021 (3)

Epithelial tumours

Thymomas

8580/3 Thymoma, NOS
8581/3 Thymoma, type A
8582/3 Thymoma, type AB
8583/3 Thymoma, type B1
8584/3 Thymoma, type B2
8585/3 Thymoma, type B3
8580/1 Micronodular thymoma with lymphoid stroma
8580/3 Metaplastic thymoma
9010/0 Lipofibroadenoma

Squamous carcinomas

8070/3 Squamous cell carcinoma, NOS
8123/3 Basaloid carcinoma
8023/3 Lymphoepithelial carcinoma

Adenocarcinomas

8140/3 Adenocarcinoma, NOS
8260/3 Low-grade papillary adenocarcinoma
8200/3 Thymic carcinoma with adenoid cystic carcinoma-like features
8144/3 Adenocarcinoma, enteric-type

Adenosquamous carcinoma

8560/3 Adenosquamous carcinoma

NUT carcinomas

8023/3 NUT carcinoma

Salivary gland-like carcinomas

8430/3 Mucoepidermoid carcinoma
8310/3 Clear cell carcinoma
8033/3 Sarcomatoid carcinoma
8980/3 Carcinosarcoma

Undifferentiated carcinoma

8020/3 Carcinoma, undifferentiated, NOS

Thymic carcinomas

8586/3 Thymic carcinoma, NOS

Thymic neuroendocrine neoplasms

Neuroendocrine tumours

8240/3 Carcinoid tumour, NOS / neuroendocrine tumour, NOS
8240/3 Typical carcinoid / neuroendocrine tumour, grade 1
8249/3 Atypical carcinoid / neuroendocrine tumour, grade 2

Neuroendocrine carcinomas

8041/3 Small cell carcinoma carcinoma

8045/3 Combined small cell carcinoma

8013/3 Large cell neuroendocrine

Appendix II: Masaoka-Koga Classification *(4)*

Stage I	Completely encapsulated tumor, macroscopically and microscopically
	- No extension to the mediastinal fat
	This group includes tumors with invasion into - but not beyond - the capsule, and tumors without capsule but without invasion of peripheral tissues.
Stage IIA	- Trans-capsular microscopic invasion ($\leq$ 3 mm, anatomo-pathological confirmation)
Stage IIB	- Macroscopic invasion in the peri-thymic fat
	- Macroscopic invasion into normal thymus or perithymic fat, confirmed on pathological examination
	- Macroscopic, non-invasive adhesions to the mediastinal pleura or pericardium. These adhesions may necessitate resection of these structures during surgery, with pathological confirmation of invasion of the perithelial fat, and of the absence of invasion of - or beyond - the mediastinal pleura or the fibrous envelope of the pericardium
Stage III	- Macroscopic extension to adjacent organs (pericardium, large vessels, lung)
	This group includes tumors with, on pathologic examination: (1) microscopic invasion of the mediastinal or visceral pleura or pericardium, or (2) direct invasion of the lung parenchyma, or (3) invasion of the phrenic or vagus nerve, confirmed on pathological examination (adhesion is not sufficient), or (4) invasion of the great vessels, confirmed on pathological examination
Stage IVA	- Tumor with pleural or pericardial implants. These grafts correspond to tumor nodules, distinct from the main tumor, with invasion of the visceral or parietal pleura, or invasion of the pericardium or epicardium.
Stage IVB	- Node metastases: anterior mediastinal, intra-thoracic, anterior or inferior cervical, or extra-thoracic
	- Hematogenous metastases
	This group includes metastases that are extra-thoracic AND outside the peri-thymic region, including lung tumors without associated pleural implants

Appendix III: Classification of neuroendocrine tumors of the thymus (WHO 2021) (3)

	Low-grade	Intermediate-grade	High-grade	
Classification of tumours with neuroendocrine morphology	Typical cacinoid	Atypical cacinoid	Large cell neuroendocrine carcinoma	Small cell carcinoma
	No necrosis < 2 mitoses/2 mm2 (mean: 1 mitosis/2 mm2)	Necrosis present (any) and/or 2-10 mitoses/2 mm2 (mean: 6.5 mitoses/2 mm2)	Non-small cell cytology Neuroendocrine markers > 10 mitoses/2 mm2 (mean: 45 mitoses/2 mm2) Frequent necrosis	Small cell cytology > 10 mitoses/2 mm2 (mean: 110 mitoses/2 mm2)

Thymic epithelial tumors: clinical aspects and positive diagnosis

Nesrine Kallel[1,3], Fatma Elloumi[2,3]

(1) Pneumology Department CHU Hédi Chaker Sfax
(2) Department of radiotherapy CHU Habib Bourguiba Sfax
(3) Faculty of Medicine of Sfax- Tunisia

Summary:

TETs occur primarily in adults between the ages of 40 and 50. In the absence of autoimmune disease, 65% of cases are discovered incidentally and 35% of cases by signs of compression or invasion of mediastinal organs.

Autoimmune manifestations are found in about one third of patients at diagnosis. Myasthenia is the most common, along with erythroblastopenia and hypogammaglobulinemia.

Diagnostic management must include both positive and differential diagnosis of an anterior mediastinal mass. Improvements in imaging techniques have improved diagnostic performance. Thoracic CT with iodinated contrast injection is considered the imaging modality of first choice in this context

The positive diagnosis of certainty is based on histological examination.

1. Introduction:

Despite being the most common etiology of adult anterior mediastinal tumors, TETs are rare (1). They are slow-growing tumors that cause few symptoms (in the absence of autoimmune disease) and are frequently discovered incidentally. In the case of associated AD (parathymic syndrome), diagnosis is easier and especially earlier (2).

2. Clinical signs:

Clinical signs are varied. At the time of diagnosis, one-third to one-half of patients are asymptomatic, with an anterior mediastinal mass found on chest radiography (3). One third of patients present with local symptoms and one third of cases are detected as part of the workup for a paraneoplastic syndrome, foremost of which is myasthenia gravis (2).

In symptomatic patients, mediastinal clinical signs are not specific.

The most frequently reported symptoms are local symptoms related to mediastinal compression (4). Chest pain, cough, and shortness of breath are present in both capsulated and invasive forms, whereas in invasive tumors, superior vena cava syndrome (SVC), hemidiaphragm paralysis (phrenic nerve involvement), and dysphonia (recurrent laryngeal nerve infiltration) are frequently observed (3,5).

Pleural effusion and chest pain are also seen if the tumor extends to the pleura (5). General signs are rarer (less than 10% of patients), and are described mainly in cases of thymic carcinoma (3).

3. Paraneoplastic syndromes:

Thymic tumors are associated with autoimmune manifestations (parathymic syndrome) in more than 20% of cases at diagnosis (4).

These "parathymic" syndromes are related to both deregulation of T cell differentiation by tumor medullary thymic epithelial cells and aberrant expression of antigens by the tumor (6).

3-1- Myasthenia :

Myasthenia gravis, an autoimmune disease related to the development of autoantibodies directed against postsynaptic acetylcholine receptors, is the most common paraneoplastic disease associated with thymoma (5).

Most series report a frequency of 30-50% in patients with thymoma, whereas only 10-15% of patients with myasthenia have a thymoma (5,7). Thymic carcinoma is rarely associated with myasthenia (5).

Like other para-thymic syndromes, the onset of myasthenia can be precessive, synchronous, or metachronous.

Myasthenia most often affects young (< 40 years) and female patients (60-70% of cases) (8).

The diagnosis is confirmed by the presence of a reversible neuromuscular block on electromyography after administration of an anticholinesterase drug (2).

Acetylcholine receptor antibody testing (positive in 90% of patients) assists in diagnosis and follow-up (2).

Myasthenia gravis is often associated with other autoimmune conditions (15% to 20% of cases), which in some series are responsible for the death of the patient in 25% of cases (6,9).

3-2- Other parathymic syndromes :

In addition to myasthenia, which occurs in approximately 30% of patients with thymoma, a multitude of paraneoplastic syndromes have been observed (Table 1). More than 25 other parathymic syndromes have been described (6) with a variable prevalence ranging from 0 to 30% depending on the series.

Of these syndromes, which occur in less than 5-10% of patients, PRCA (10% of cases) and hypogammaglobulinemia (5-10% of cases) (6,7) are the most common syndromes.

Very rarely, thymic carcinomas have been found to be associated with polymyositis, dermatomyositis or erythrocytosis (10).

Neuroendocrine thymic tumors are frequently associated with endocrinopathies (up to 30% of cases), including Cushing's syndrome, multiple endocrine neoplasia type 1 (NEM-1 or Wermer's syndrome), and growth hormone hyper-secretion (GHRH) with acromegaly (5).

4. Positive diagnosis:

Diagnostic management should include both positive and differential diagnosis of an anterior mediastinal mass.

The diagnosis of thymic tumors is usually suspected clinically based largely on the CT scan appearance of an anterior mediastinal mass (7). Clinical examination may reveal signs related to an associated parathymic syndrome or local invasion (CVS syndrome) (5). The positive diagnosis of certainty is based on histological examination (2).

The first step in dealing with a mediastinal lesion suspected of being a thymic epithelial tumor is to establish the differential diagnosis with other anterior mediastinal tumors and nonmalignant thymic lesions (4).

Chest CT with iodinated contrast injection is considered the imaging modality of first choice in this setting ((4,5,11). MRI is of little use in the diagnosis of thymic malignancies, except in cases of suspected infiltration of the heart and stomach (5,12).

PET has been evaluated in its ability to differentiate thymic hyperplasia from thymoma, low-risk versus high-risk thymoma, and thymoma versus thymic carcinoma (5).

Improvements in imaging techniques have improved diagnostic performance and reduced the need for biopsy (1).

The anatomopathological diagnosis of certainty is most often surgical; it can sometimes be provided by simple percutaneous puncture (1,13).

The need for pre-therapeutic biopsy also depends on the resectability of the tumor (4). Small "typical" encapsulated thymomas are excised up front for diagnosis and treatment. Large invasive and "atypical" thymomas are best managed by biopsy to ascertain the histology of the tumor and to assess its invasive potential. However, there is general agreement that biopsy should be reserved for undefined chest CT findings that may suggest lymphoma, or for unresectable tumors prior to induction chemotherapy or definitive chemoradiotherapy (5,14). This approach has gained acceptance because of the long-standing dictum that preoperative biopsy should be avoided for fear of local implantation.

The standard approach is an anterior mediastinotomy. Mediastinoscopy is not recommended, because this approach allows access to the middle compartment rather than the anterior mediastinum. Needle cytopuncture is also not recommended (6,7).

References:

1. A. Ouabdelmoumen AS, F. Naciri, Z. Dehbi, Z. Bourhaleb, M. Elhfid, L. Mezouar. Multimodal treatment of thymic epithelial tumors. Journal of Functional Ventilation and Pulmonology. 2015;6(19):39-43.

2	Perrotin C, Régnard JF. Tumours of the thymus. EMC - Pneumology. 2005;2(1):1-12.

Nicolas Girard FoM, Paul Van Houtte, Jean-Franc¸ois Cordier, and Paul van Schil. Thymoma A Focus on Current Therapeutic Management. Journal of Thoracic Oncology. 2009;4.

4	Girard N, du Vignaux CM, Besse B, Rythmic. Thymic tumours. Journal of Respiratory Diseases News. 2016;8(5):457-71.

5	Enrico Ruffini FV. Management of thymic tumors: a European perspective. Journal of Thoracic Disease. 2014;6.

6.	N. Girard BB, RYTHMIC. Updates in the management of thymoma and thymic carcinoma. La Lettre du Pneumologue. 2012.

7	Charles R. Thomas J, Cameron D. Wright, and Patrick J. Loehrer, Sr. Thymoma State of the Art. Journal of Clinical Oncology. 1999:2280-9.

Ruffié P G-DG, Fervers B, Lehmann M, Regnard JF, Resbeut M. Standards, options and recommendations for the management of patients with thymus epithelial tumours. Bull Cancer. 1999;86:365-84.

9.	Evoli A LE. Paraneoplastic Disorders in Thymoma Patients. J Thoac Oncol. 2014;9.

10.	Inoue Y TL, Martins RG.. Thymic carcinoma associated with paraneoplastic polymyositis. J Clin Oncol. 2009;27.

11.	Ruffini E OA, Novero D,. Neuroendocrine tumors of the thymus. Thorac Surg Clin. 2011;21:13-23.

12.	EM. M. Advances in thymoma imaging. J Thorac

Imaging. 2013;28:69-80.

13.	Jacot W QX, Pujo JL. . Treatment of thymic epithelial tumors Toward multidisciplinary management. Rev Mal Respir. 2006;23.

14.	Detterbeck FC PA. Surg Thymic tumors. Ann Thorac. 2004;77:1860-9.

Radiological aspects of thymic epithelial tumors
Basma Souissi[1,2], Anis Moalla[1,2]

1- Radiology Department CHU Hbib Bourguiba Sfax

2- Faculty of Medicine of Sfax

Summary:

Thymomas account for 20% of anterior mediastinal tumors and are accompanied by myasthenia in 30-50% of cases. Surgical treatment allows a clear clinical improvement. Therefore, the role of imaging, based essentially on CT scan, is essential to guide the therapeutic attitude by looking for the criteria of resectability of thymomas. The CT/MRI pairing also allows the differential diagnosis with thymic hyperplasia and thymic carcinoma, which require treatment with chemotherapy.

I- Introduction:

Thymomas account for 20% of tumors of the anterior mediastinum in adults [1,2] and are the second most common cause of myasthenia gravis, after thymic hyperplasia, which is found in 15 to 20% of patients [3].

Therefore, the role of imaging is essential to differentiate between thymoma and thymic hyperplasia on the one hand, and to select patients for surgery on the other. Since the discovery of an upper mediastinal tumour may be fortuitous on a standard X-ray or a thoracic CT scan performed for another indication [4], in the case of myasthenia gravis, thoracic CT is the first-line examination.

II- Chest X-ray:

Standard radiography, although it has no place in the characterization of thymomas, allows the positive and topographic diagnosis of an anterior mediastinal mass as well as an etiologic approach. Indeed, it shows a homogeneous mediastinal opacity, with a clear external boundary convex to the lung parenchyma and an internal boundary embedded in the mediastinum that erases the edge of the heart. Applying the silhouette sign, this opacity is of anterior mediastinal topography (Fig1) of which tumors of thymic origin are the most frequent [4]. Thus, for a better characterization of this opacity, a thoracic CT scan is required.

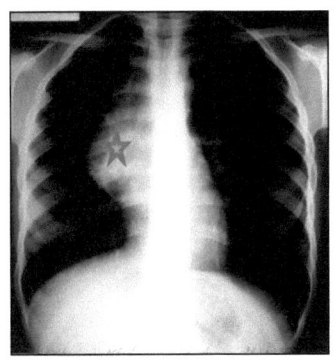

Fig1: Frontal thoracic radiograph of a 35-year-old man who presented with myasthenia gravis: homogeneous mediastinal opacity erasing the right edge of the heart ( ) of anterior topography with the silhouette sign.

III- Contribution of thoracic computed tomography (:

Computed tomography (CT), performed without and after injection of contrast medium, is the examination of choice for the diagnosis, characterization and extension of thymic tumors [5,6]. It typically shows a round or oval mass in the anterior mediastinum, often lateralized, with homogeneous or heterogeneous enhancement after injection of contrast medium [7] and may contain calcifications (Fig. 2).

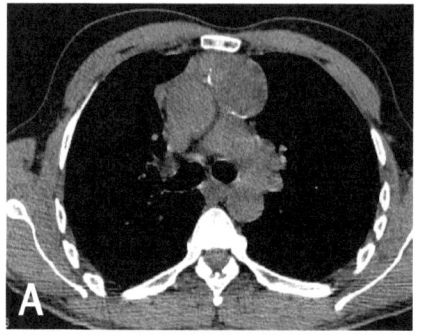 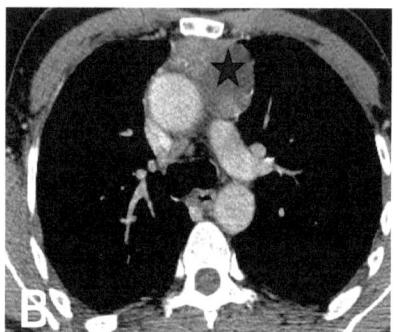

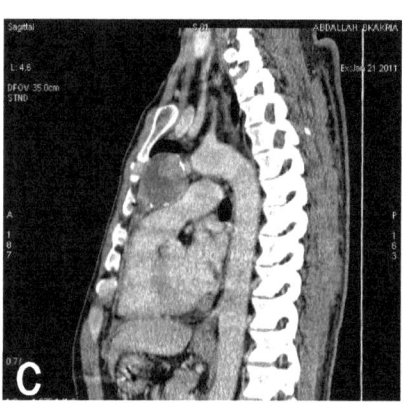
Fig2: Chest CT in axial sections (A) without injection, (B) with injection; (C) sagittal section after injection: anterior mediastinal mass, rounded in density and heterogeneous in enhancement, containing areas of necrosis and peripheral calcifications. Pathology: intermediate grade thymoma

CT can also differentiate between a thymoma and focal thymus hyperplasia as a homogeneous mass that respects the shape of the thymus and contains fatty areas [8].

IV- Contribution of magnetic resonance imaging (MRI) :

MRI, performed as a second-line procedure in some cases to eliminate differential diagnoses, includes T1- and T2-weighted double inversion-recovery axial sequences, T2-weighted sagittal sequences with fat saturation, axial phase and phase opposition sequences, axial diffusion sequence, gradient echo sequence, and T1 axial sequences with injection of Gadolinium [8]. It shows an anterior mediastinal mass with intermediate T1 and T2 signal superior to that of the muscles and without signal drop after fat saturation [8] and without signal drop on the opposite phase sequence compared with the ophase sequence, unlike thymic hyperplasia.

However, the role of imaging is essential in the therapeutic decision by looking for the criteria of complete resection, which is a prognostic factor for thymomas [9,10]. Indeed, a circumscribed mass with clear contours, homogeneous without hemorrhagic or necrotic changes and without signs of extension may be completely resectable even for intermediate grade lesions (WHO type B2 and B3) [11] without the need for MRI.

On the other hand, CT can evoke the diagnosis of invasive thymoma or thymic carcinoma requiring chemotherapy, in front of a mass of irregular contours, heterogeneous containing necrotic or cystic remodeling, mediastinal adenomegaly with signs of fat or vessel invasion: circumference encompassing at least 180°, occlusion with intimate tumor-vessel contact [12,13]. In addition to these findings, MRI due to its better contrast resolution, can demonstrate a peripheral capsule or septations, in favor of the diagnosis of thymoma [12]. In the absence of discriminatory criteria, a biopsy under CT control is appropriate for anatomopathological diagnosis.

Another discriminating criterion between thymoma and thymic carcinoma is the potential for locoregional dissemination of thymomas, especially pleural metastases, and the higher risk of extra-thoracic dissemination of thymic carcinomas [4].

References:

1. Strollo DC, Rosado-de-Christenson ML, Jett JR. Primary mediastinal tumors. Part I: tumors of the anterior mediastinum. Chest 1997;112:511e22.

2. Takahashi K, Al-Janabi NJ. Computed tomography and magnetic resonance imaging of mediastinal tumors. J Magn Reson Imaging2010;32:1325e39.

3. Onodera H. The role of the thymus in the pathogenesis of myasthenia gravis. Tohoku J Exp Med. 2005;207(2):87-98.

4. J.-Y. Gaubert, F. Cohen, V. Vidal et al. Imaging of mediastinal tumors. Revue de Pneumologie clinique (2010) 66, 17-27

5. Marom EM, Rosado-de-Christenson ML, Bruzzi JF, et al. Standard report terms for chest computed tomography reports of anterior mediastinal masses suspicious for thymoma. J Thorac Oncol 2011;6:S1717e23.

6. Ruffini E, Filosso PL, Lausi P, et al. Thymic tumors. In: Stahel RA, editor. Lung cancer therapy annual 7. London: Informa Healthcare; 2012. pp. 151e70.

7. Takahashi K, Al-Janabi NJ. Computed tomography and magnetic resonance imaging of mediastinal tumors. J Magn Reson Imaging. 2010;32(6):1325-1339.

8. Phung Anh Tuan, Mai Van Vien, Hoang Van Dong et al. The Value of CT and MRI for Determining Thymoma in Patients With Myasthenia Gravis. Cancer Control. 2019; Volume 26: 1-10

9. Kondo K, Monden Y. Therapy for thymic epothelial tumors, a clinical study of 1320 patients from Japan. Ann Thor Surg 2003;76:878-85.

10. Strobel P, Bauer A, Puppe B, Kraushaar T, Krein A, Toyka K, et al. Tumor recurrence and survival in patients treated for thymomas and thymic squamous cell carcinomas. A retrospective analysis. J Clin Oncol 2004;22:1501-9.

11. Travis WD, Brambilla E, Müller-Hermelink HK, Harris CC. WHO classification of tumors. pathology and genetics of tumors of the lung, pleura, thymus and heart. Lyon: IARC Press; 2004.

12. Sadohara J, Fujimoto K, Muller NL, Kato S, Takamori S, Ohkuma K, et al. Thymic epithelial tumors: comparison of CT and MR imaging findings of low-risk thymomas, high-risk thymomas, and thymic carcinomas. Eur J Radiol 2006;60:70-9.

13. Tomiyama N, Honda O, Tsubamoto M, Inoue A, Sumikawa H, Kuriyama K, et al. Anterior mediastinal tumors: diagnostic accuracy of CT and MRI. Eur J Radiol 2009;69:280-8.

Minimally invasive surgery for thymoma: indications and approach

Zied Chaari ; Abdessalem Hentati ; Walid Abid ; Imed Frikha

University of Sfax - Department of Thoracic and Cardiovascular Surgery CHU Habib Bourguiba Sfax - Tunisia

Summary:

Surgery has an important place in the treatment of mediastinal tumors, particularly thymomas whether or not associated with myasthenia gravis. Minimally invasive techniques have gained ground since 1990 and are increasingly an essential approach for the resection of mediastinal and thymic tumours. We present the different possible minimally invasive approaches for thymoma surgery, their variants, and the surgical outcomes associated with this surgery.

I- Introduction:

Surgery has an important place in the treatment of mediastinal tumors, especially thymomas, whether or not they are associated with myasthenia gravis. For a long time, these tumors were mainly treated by sternotomy or thoracotomy [1,2].

Minimally invasive techniques have gained ground since 1990 and are increasingly an essential approach for the resection of mediastinal and thymic tumors.

II- Minimally invasive approaches for thymoma surgery:

II-1- Mini sternotomy :

This is a minimally invasive surgery, with an incision from the sternal fork to the third or fourth intercostal space. The opening of the sternal manubrium alone (manubriotomy) may be sufficient to approach and resect the entire thymus gland in its compartment. However, some authors state that manubriotomy does not represent a minimally invasive approach [3].

II-2- Cervicotomy :

The patient is intubated with a selective tube. The patient is installed in dorsal decubitus with a log under the shoulder blades and the head in slight hyperextension. The scope is wide, from the mandible to the umbilicus. During the cervical phase, the surgeon is positioned at the patient's head, and during the subxiphoid phase on the patient's right. Placement of a retractor under the sternal manubrium would allow upward sternal traction with better exposure to the anterior mediastinum. This approach has been used by surgical teams with or without sternal suspension [4].

II-3- Video-assisted thoracic surgery (VATS) :

It is an option to access lesions in the inferior, posterior and anterior mediastinum. It is performed under general anaesthesia and requires selective intubation to exclude the lung and provide sufficient working space. This approach is based on the principle of using a single or multiple trocars, a rigid optic with or without angulation (0° or 30° or 45° optic), with a mini thoracic incision and a slight rib spread using a Tuffier retractor.

II-4-Exclusive videothoracoscopy (VTS) :

It is currently (along with VATS) the most commonly used approach for thymic resection [5,6]. The procedure is performed under general anesthesia with selective intubation. The patient is in lateral decubitus position. This approach is based on the principle of three triangulated trocars introduced through parietal openings between 5 and 10 mm in diameter. The lower trocar is used for the optics and the lateral trocar to introduce the specific endoscopic instruments. The surgical procedure is monitored on the monitor placed in front of the surgeon.

II-5-Robotic Assisted Thoracic Surgery (RATS) :

RATS was introduced to overcome the difficulties of VTS. It is currently widely adopted in the treatment of anterior mediastinal tumors with instruments that can articulate with 7 degrees of freedom, allowing safe dissection around vascular and nerve structures and for tiny masses and hard-to-reach anatomical areas, such as the anterior mediastinum. This is a new technique using robotic arms inserted through the chest wall with the surgeon controlling from a distance. Using a console and a three-dimensional stereoscopic system, the surgeon operates with the same visual rapport as in open surgery. Thanks to the robot, the surgeon operates through reduced incisions without compromising the dexterity and precision of his natural gestures. The natural tremors of the surgeon's hand are eliminated by an electronic filtering system that ensures stable and predictable control of the instruments.

II-6- Uniportal VATS :

This technique is based on the same principles as videothoracoscopy, but with the use of a single mini-incision to approach the thorax (Figure 1). Through this single incision, all the instruments necessary for surgical removal are introduced, before extracting the surgical specimen.

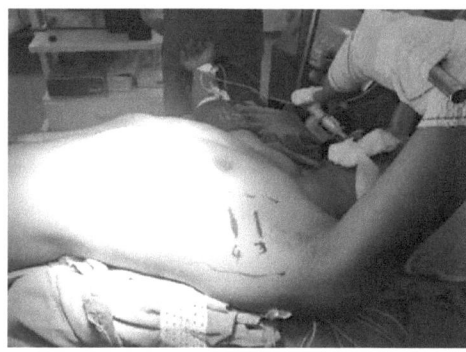

Figure 1: Thymectomy set-up using the left Uniportal approach

III- Surgical variants of minimally invasive approaches:

Regardless of the approach used, the surgical procedure should provide the most radical resection possible (in the presence of a thymic tumor or without a thymic tumor in myasthenia gravis). The best surgical approach should include an approach to both pleural cavities, as well as the lower cervical area down to the level of the thyroid gland [7].

Other than the cervical, trans-sternal, or thoracic approach (uni or bilateral), the subxiphoid approach for thymic resections has been described and adopted by many surgical teams [8-10]

A hybrid approach associating two or more surgical techniques and/or approaches has been described. Indeed, a double cervical and subxiphoid approach can be used to perform extended thymectomies to the mediastinal fat, or to other mediastinal structures such as the pericardium. This procedure can be facilitated by sternal suspension throughout the operation [4].

Several experiences and surgical variants have been described in minimally invasive thymic resection such as:

- The use of a single uniportal approach via the trans-cervical route[11]
- The coupling: videothoracoscopy with cervical approach [12]
- The use of a double uniportal thoracic approach[13]
- The use of a uniportal approach on one side of the chest and a multi-portal approach on the other [14].

Minimally invasive thymic resections can be performed by the right approach [15] (which is the most commonly used approach allowing work to be carried out at a distance from the left heart and better control of the left inominate venous trunk), by the left approach (ensuring better control and visibility of the left phrenic nerve), or by the bilateral approach [13] (with the patient in the supine position allowing either a double approach by videothoracoscopy, or a single approach by the cervical or supra xyphoid approach). The latter, described as a "comfort" approach, would allow a better radical exeresis [7].

No significant difference in terms of operative time, blood loss, postoperative drainage time and hospitalization was noted when comparing the intercostal and subxiphoid routes [16].

IV- Indications for minimally invasive surgery:

The thymus plays a central role in the development of the immune system in the pre- and early post-natal period. However, during life, all possible components of the thymus can be reactivated (in a physiological or pathological way) and therefore be responsible for many pathologies whether benign or malignant, tumoral or not, or autoimmune or not.

Myasthenia gravis is the main indication for thymic resection (thymectomy) with extended removal of all mediastinal fat (Figure 2).

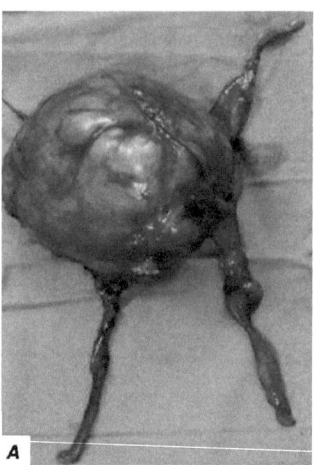

Figure 2: Thymoma surgical specimen

The latter could contain ectopic thymic tissue responsible for the perpetuation of muscle fatigability even after resection of the thymus alone. Minimally invasive surgery has been described as the preferred approach for this condition.

Other surgical indications have been proposed for minimally invasive thymic resection:

- The presence of a tumor of the thymic lodge, whether or not associated with myasthenia gravis.
- Presence of a non-invasive thymic tumor (stage I and II)
- The presence of an invasive thymic tumor (stage III or even stage IV)
- A thymic tumor size of less than 5 cm.

However, other indications for minimally invasive surgery have been reported depending on the approach used, tumor size, stage and extent of surgical removal (Table I).

Table I: Surgical approaches and indications for thymectomies

Authors	Year	Number	Minimally invasive approach (%)	Indications
Migliore et al[17]	2017	13	Cervicotomy (100)	MG without thymic tumor Size < 2cm
Suda et al[8]	2020	147	Uniportal subxiphoid (100)	MG with or without thymoma Thymoma stages I or II Size: 0.5 - 17cm
Hida et al[6]	2012	51	VATS (100)	Size < 7cm Cystic lesion with wall < 5mm
Wang et al [18]	2019	103	VATS right (21)	MG with or without thymoma Thymoma stage I or II or III Non-invasive thymoma on TVI
Marulli et al[1919]	2012	79	RATS left (82.4) RATS right (12.6) RATS bilateral (5)	Thymoma stage I or II Size < 12cm
Marulli et al[20]	2016	134	RATS left (38) RATS right (59.8) RATS bilateral (2.2)	MG with or without thymoma Thymoma stages I, II, III or IV Size < 10cm
Miyata et al[21]	2019	17	VATS (82.3) RATS (17.7)	Thymic carcinomas Neuroendocrine carcinoma stage I or II
Ishibashi et al[22]	2012	33	VATS (36)	MG with or without solid or cystic tumor Non-invasive thymoma Size < 6cm
Matsumura et al [23]	2006	50	VATS (100)	Benign thymic lesions Non-invasive thymoma (stage I, II without TVI invasion) Size < 5cm
Matsumoto et al[24]	2012	27	VATS (74) VTS + sternal elevation (11)	MG associated or not with a non-invasive thymoma

					Benign thymic pathology
					Size < 5cm
Kimura et al [25]	2013	74		VATS (61)	Thymoma stage I or II
					Thymoma without capsular rupture
					Size < 5cm

VATS: video-assisted thoracic surgery / RATS: robot-assisted thoracic surgery / VTS: video thoracoscopy / MG: Myasthenia Gravis

V- Results of minimally invasive surgery:

Minimally invasive thymic surgery is correlated with morbidity rates ranging from 1.8 to 17% and mortality rates between 0 and 6%.

The most frequently reported complications after minimally invasive thymic surgery are:

- Complete atrial fibrillation arrhythmia (CAFA)
- Myasthenic seizures (especially in cases of thymoma associated with myasthenia gravis).
- Postoperative pleural effusions (pneumothorax or postoperative pleurisy).
- Lung or surgical site infections
- Postoperative hemothorax that may require revision surgery
- Embolic accidents: mainly pulmonary embolism.
- Phrenic nerve injuries[24]

In a series of 2835 patients operated by VATS or median sternotomy for thymoma, no significant difference was observed between the two groups of patients in terms of morbidity, quality of surgical excision, overall survival and even in terms of 5-year recurrence-free survival [26].

A meta-analysis of 1222 patients operated on for stage I and II thymoma concluded that VATS is associated with less blood loss, shorter drainage time and hospital stay [27].

When comparing the three approaches to thymectomy (open, minimally invasive VATS and RATS), in a series including 1223 thymectomies, the minimally invasive approach was associated with a shorter hospital stay than open surgery [28]. No significant difference between these groups was observed in terms of quality of resection, readmission rate, mortality and long-term survival.

Another study comparing VATS and RATS for the treatment of stage I thymoma showed the superiority of RATS with a less invasive procedure, a shorter drainage period and a shorter hospital stay than VATS. However, RATS was significantly more expensive [29].

The recurrence rate of thymoma after robotic resection varies between 0 and 11% [30]. The different characteristics of VATS and RATS have been summarized in Table II :

Table II: Comparison between the different approaches for thymectomy

Comparison	Open surgery - VATS [27]	VATS - RATS [29]
Benefits	- ↓ muscle section - ↓ bone fractures - ↓ pain - ↓ blood loss - ↓ drainage time - ↓ length of stay - Best recovery	- Less invasive procedure - ↓ drainage period - ↓ length of stay
Disadvantages		More expensive RATS

VATS: video-assisted thoracic surgery / RATS: robot-assisted thoracic surgery

Variations of the surgical technique and approach used in RATS surgery have been reported in a series of 110 patients who underwent robotic thymectomy via the subxiphoid approach with favorable postoperative outcomes (morbidity at 1.8%) and a mean hospital stay of 2.2 days +/- 1.4 days [31].

Therefore, thymectomy by RATS has been associated with an overall 5-year survival of 100% for thymoma and 95% for thymic carcinoma with an estimated 5-year recurrence-free survival of 94% for thymoma [32].

The 10-year survival rate for all stages combined is 76% for complete resection. This long-term survival rate drops to 26% in case of incomplete resection [33] or advanced histological stage (from 100% for stage I to 25% for stage IV). Despite a well-conducted surgical treatment, the recurrence rate of encapsulated thymoma is 2% to 12% of cases [34].

Table III reports the surgical results of thymectomies according to the minimally invasive approaches used in the literature.

Table III: Minimally invasive thymectomy surgical series

Authors	Year	Number	Thymoma (%)	Minimally invasive approaches (%)	Morbidity (%)	Mortality (%)	Survival at 5 years
Wright et al[5]	2002	26	**3,7**	VATS (100)	3,8	0	--
Petkov et al[35]	2004	232	**28.4**	Cervicotomy (19.8) Sternal suspension (66.8)	--	0.92	94%
Jurado et al[36]	2012	139	**66**	VATS (22.3)	9,1	0	--
Agatsuma et al[26]	2017	2835	**100**	VATS (9.9)	9.3 5.7	--	--
Yang et al[28]	2020	1223	**100**	VATS (11) RATS (15)	< 10 < 10	< 10 < 10	89.4%
Luzzi et al[37]	2020	114	**100**	RATS (50)	12 9	4 2	--
Kang et al[32]	2020	158	**84**	RATS (100)	4.4	0	--
Kang et al[31]	2020	110	**60.9**	RATS under Xyphoid (100)	1.8	0	--
Marulli et al[20]	2016	134	**100**	RATS right (59.8) left (38) and bilateral (2.2)	17.1 **Pleural recurrence (0.7%)**	--	97%
Miyata et al[21]	2019	17	**0 (carcinomas)**	VATS (82.3) RATS (17.7)	6	0	84.4%
Pupovac et al[38]	2020	17	**100**	Uniportal VATS	--	0	100%
Suda et al[39]	2020	147	**49.6**	Uniportal subxiphoid	4	0	--

VATS: video-assisted thoracic surgery, RATS: robot-assisted thoracic surgery

References:

1. Dosios, T., E. Kouskos, and V. Kyriakou, *Surgical management of mediastinal lesions.* Tuberk Toraks, 2006. **54**(3): p. 207-12.
2. Bacha, E.A., et al. *surgery for invasive primary mediastinal tumors.* Ann Thorac Surg, 1998. **66**(1): p. 234-9.
3. Zieliński, M., *Definitions and standard indications of minimally-invasive techniques in thymic surgery.* J Vis Surg, 2017. **3**(99): p. 99.
4. Takeo, S., T. Sakada, and T. Yano, *Video-assisted extended thymectomy in patients with thymoma by lifting the sternum.* Ann Thorac Surg, 2001. **71**(5): p. 1721-3.
5. Wright, G.M., S. Barnett, and C.P. Clarke, *Video-assisted thoracoscopic thymectomy for myasthenia gravis.* Intern Med J, 2002. **32**(8): p. 367-71.
6. Hida, Y., et al, *[Indication of video-assisted thoracic surgery for mediastinal mass lesions].* Kyobu Geka, 2012. **65**(11): p. 934-8.
7. Zieliński, M., *Surgical Approaches to Myasthenia Gravis: Perspective of Anatomy and Radicality in Surgery.* Thorac Surg Clin, 2019. **29**(2): p. 159-164.
8. Suda, T., *Uniportal subxiphoid video-assisted thoracoscopic thymectomy.* J Vis Surg, 2016. **2**(123): p. 123.
9. Zieliński, M., et al, *Subxiphoid uniportal VATS thymectomy.* J Vis Surg, 2017. **3**(171): p. 171.
10. Liu, Z., R. Yang, and Y. Sun, *Non-intubated subxiphoid uniportal video-assisted thoracoscopic thymectomy.* Interact Cardiovasc Thorac Surg, 2019. **29**(5): p. 742-745.
11. Lemaître, P.H. and S. Keshavjee, *Uniportal Video-Assisted Transcervical Thymectomy.* Thorac Surg Clin, 2019. **29**(2): p. 187-194.
12. Novellino, L., et al, *"Extended" thymectomy, without sternotomy, performed by cervicotomy and thoracoscopic technique in the treatment of myasthenia gravis.* Int Surg, 1994. **79**(4): p. 378-81.
13. Caronia, F.P., et al, *Uniportal bilateral video-assisted sequential thoracoscopic extended thymectomy.* J Vis Surg, 2017. **3**(69): p. 69.
14. Infante, M., et al. *VATS thymectomy for early stage thymoma and myasthenia gravis: combined right-sided uniportal and left-sided three-portal approach.* J Vis Surg, 2017. **3**(144): p. 144.
15. Ooi, A. and M. Sibayan, *Uniportal video assisted thoracoscopic surgery thymectomy (right approach).* J Vis Surg, 2016. **2**(13): p. 13.
16. Liu, Z. and R. Yang, *Comparison of Subxiphoid and Intercostal Uniportal Thoracoscopic Thymectomy for Nonmyasthenic Early-Stage Thymoma: A Retrospective Single-Center Propensity-Score Matching Analysis.* Thorac Cardiovasc Surg, 2021. **69**(2): p. 173-180.
17. Migliore, M., et al, *Single incision extended video assisted transcervical thymectomy.* J Vis Surg, 2017. **3**(154): p. 154.
18. Wang, G.W., et al. *comparison between thoracoscopic and open approaches in thymoma resection.* J Thorac Dis, 2019. **11**(10): p. 4159-4168.

19. Marulli, G., et al. *robot-aided thoracoscopic thymectomy for early-stage thymoma: a multicenter European study.* J Thorac Cardiovasc Surg, 2012. **144**(5): p. 1125-30.
20. Marulli, G., et al, *Multi-institutional European experience of robotic thymectomy for thymoma.* Ann Cardiothorac Surg, 2016. **5**(1): p. 18-25.
21. Miyata, R., et al, *Survival outcomes after minimally invasive thymectomy for early-stage thymic carcinoma.* Surg Today, 2019. **49**(4): p. 357-360.
22. Ishibashi, H. and K. Okubo, *[Surgery for mediastinal tumor; by video-assisted thoracoscopic thymo-thymomectomy with sternal lifting].* Kyobu Geka, 2012. **65**(11): p. 969-72.
23. Matsumura, Y. and T. Kondo, *[Indication and procedure of video-assisted thoracoscopic surgery to thymic disease].* Kyobu Geka, 2006. **59**(8 Suppl): p. 742-8.
24. Matsumoto, K., et al, *[Minimally invasive surgery for thymic disease].* Kyobu Geka, 2012. **65**(11): p. 955-9.
25. Kimura, T., et al, *The oncological feasibility and limitations of video-assisted thoracoscopic thymectomy for early-stage thymomas.* Eur J Cardiothorac Surg, 2013. **44**(3): p. e214-8.
26. Agatsuma, H., et al, *Video-Assisted Thoracic Surgery Thymectomy Versus Sternotomy Thymectomy in Patients With Thymoma.* Ann Thorac Surg, 2017. **104**(3): p. 1047-1053.
27. Rusidanmu, A., et al, *Trans-sternotomy versus video-assisted thoracic surgery for early-stage thymoma patients: a meta-analysis.* Gland Surg, 2020. **9**(2): p. 342-351.
28. Yang, C.J., et al, *A national analysis of open versus minimally invasive thymectomy for stage I to III thymoma.* J Thorac Cardiovasc Surg, 2020. **160**(2): p. 555-567 e15.
29. Ye, B., et al. *Video-assisted thoracoscopic surgery versus robotic-assisted thoracoscopic surgery in the surgical treatment of Masaoka stage I thymoma.* World J Surg Oncol, 2013. **11**(157): p. 157.
30. Rueckert, J., et al, *Robotic-assisted thymectomy: surgical procedure and results.* Thorac Cardiovasc Surg, 2015. **63**(3): p. 194-200.
31. Kang, C.H., et al. *the robotic thymectomy via the subxiphoid approach: technique and early outcomes.* Eur J Cardiothorac Surg, 2020. **58**(Suppl_1): p. i39-i43.
32. Kang, C.H., et al, *Long-Term Outcomes of Robotic Thymectomy in Patients With Thymic Epithelial Tumors.* Ann Thorac Surg, 2020. **29**(20): p. 31817-8.
33. Regnard, J.F., et al, *Prognostic factors and long-term results after thymoma resection: a series of 307 patients.* J Thorac Cardiovasc Surg, 1996. **112**(2): p. 376-84.
34. Strollo, D.C., M.L. Rosado de Christenson, and J.R. Jett, *Primary mediastinal tumors. Part 1: tumors of the anterior mediastinum.* Chest, 1997. **112**(2): p. 511-22.
35. Petkov, R., et al, *[Thymectomy for myastenia gravis: 25-year experience].* Khirurgiia (Sofiia), 2004. **60**(3): p. 27-9.
36. Jurado, J., et al. *minimally invasive thymectomy and open thymectomy: outcome analysis of 263 patients.* Ann Thorac Surg, 2012. **94**(3): pp. 974-81; discussion 981-2.
37. Luzzi, L., et al, *Robotic surgery vs. open surgery for thymectomy, a retrospective case-match study.* J Robot Surg, 2021. **15**(3): p. 375-379.
38. Pupovac, S.S., et al. *Intermediate oncologic outcomes after uniportal video-assisted thoracoscopic thymectomy for early-stage thymoma.* J Thorac Dis, 2020. **12**(8): p. 4025-4032.

39. Suda, T., et al, *Early outcomes in 147 consecutive cases of subxiphoid single-port thymectomy and evaluation of learning curves.* Eur J Cardiothorac Surg, 2020. **58**(Suppl_1): p. i44-i49.

Surgery for locally invasive thymomas

Zied Chaari ; Abdessalem Hentati ; Walid Abid ; Imed Frikha

University of Sfax - Department of Thoracic and Cardiovascular Surgery CHU Habib Bourguiba Sfax - Tunisia

Summary:

Thymomas are the most frequent tumours of the anterior mediastinum, the prognosis of which depends closely on the histological classification, the Masaoka classification and the quality of excision. Surgical excision consists of a complete resection of the thymus (thymectomy) extended to the invaded structures that may involve the mediastinal vessels, the lung, the phrenic nerves, or the cardiac cavities. The possible approaches are variable and include open and minimally invasive surgery. The results and postoperative complications are variable depending on the series and the invaded structures resected.

I- Definition:

Thymomas represent the most common tumors of the anterior mediastinum with more than 50% of all anterior tumors [1]. Invasive thymomas can be defined as tumors of the thymic cavity with microscopic or macroscopic capsule invasion (Masaoka Coga stage II), invasion of adjacent structures (Masaoka stage III: including pleural, pericardial, or vascular involvement), or with nodular pericardial, pleural, or distant dissemination (pulmonary nodules, lymph node involvement, or other distant organs). The prognosis depends closely on the histological classification, the Masaoka classification and the quality of excision, which must be as complete as possible, even for advanced stages [2].

II-Procedures used :

For a long time, surgical excision of invasive thymic tumors has been performed via a median sternotomy [3,4]. This approach allows excellent exposure of the entire anterior mediastinum with good approach to various adjacent invasive structures [5].

Other open approaches are possible, such as sternotomy coupled with an anterior thoracotomy (Hemi clamshell approach) [6], or the use of a double anterior thoracotomy associated with a transverse sternotomy (Clamshell).

With the advent of minimally invasive surgical techniques, several variants of surgical approach have been described and used by several teams. Indeed, video-assisted thoracic surgery or VATS (despite being currently the standard approach for thymic resections for myasthenias with or without stage I thymic tumor), is increasingly used as an approach for the resection of invasive stage II, stage III thymic tumors or even for the treatment of thymic carcinomas [7,8].

Robot-assisted thoracic surgery (RATS) can also be used for the treatment of invasive thymic tumors [7]. The excellent endothoracic vision, the better dexterity of the robotic arms ensuring 360° rotation and movements, the possibility of using CO_2 insufflation intraoperatively for more working space, the precision of the gestures performed with a significant reduction of tremors and parasitic movements, have made RATS an unavoidable approach for enlarged thymic resections in a narrow thoracic area.

Other variants of minimally invasive surgery have also been described for invasive thymic tumor resection such as video thoracoscopy (VATS), robotic-assisted thoracic surgery (RATS) [9], or the use of a bilateral double thoracic VATS approach [8].

Extensive thymic resection can also be performed via a minimally invasive approach with a single incision (Uniportal VATS) via the thoracic or subxiphoid approach [10,11].

III-Possible extensions of surgical excisions :

The principle of carcinologic resection surgery is to perform a complete removal of the tumor as well as the invaded structures, while having safe margins in the healthy zone and microscopically healthy boundaries (R0 resection). The presence of microscopically affected (R1 resection) or macroscopically invaded (R2 resection) boundaries are factors signifying failure of radical surgical treatment [12].

Therefore, the extension of surgical excision in cases of invasive thymic tumors involve, in addition to complete thymic resection (thymectomy), an extended excision to the various adjacent invaded structures and may include:

- Mediastinal fat most often invaded in capsular invasion (stage II)
- The mediastinal pleura or pleural cavity[13,14]
- Pericardium: Tumor extension outside the thymic capsule to the pericardium is the most frequent indication for extended resection of the pericardium in monobloc with thymectomy. This resection may be on a limited area, or extended to a large part of the pericardium responsible for a significant exposure of the heart. In this case, pericardial reconstruction using patches, non-resorbable sutures, or plates is necessary in order to avoid cardiac torsion and dislocation (Figure 1).

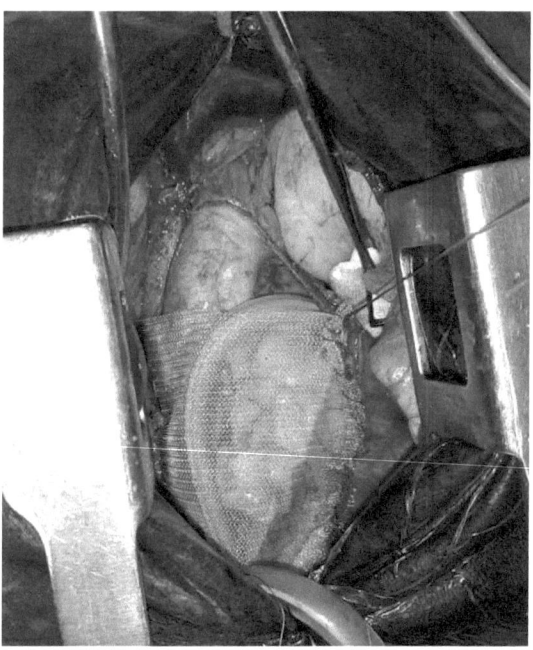

Figure 1: Extended thymectomy to the pericardium and left phrenic nerve with pericardial reconstruction using a propylene plate

- The phrenic nerve(s): Whatever the technique and the approach used, preservation of the phrenic nerves as far as possible should be the surgeon's priority, especially in the case of associated myasthenia gravis. Indeed, because of the often associated alveolar hypoventilation, phrenic nerve damage would worsen the respiratory status postoperatively. Phrenic nerve damage is observed in about 7% of thymic surgeries [15]. The intraoperative use of phrenic stimulators allows more accurate detection of the limits of excision near the phrenic nerves [16].
- The lung (Figure 2): ranging from simple atypical resection (wedge resection) to a regulated anatomical resection (lobectomy or even a pneumonectomy) [17].

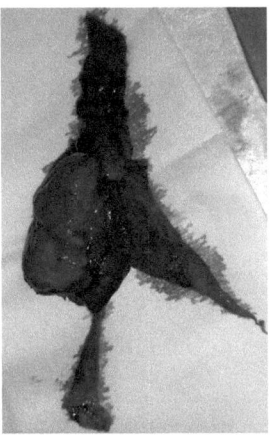

Figure 2: Extended right upper lobe thymectomy (atypical right upper lobe wedge resection) with single block resection

- Vessels: which may include:
  o *Mediastinal venous structures*: on the inominate venous trunk [18] (treated by simple ligation or by venous bypasses), or the superior vena cava (partial resection with clamping and lateral vascular suture without or with vascular or pericardial patch [19,20], or complete resection with prosthetic replacement [21,22]).

  In the case of a procedure on the vena cava or the inominate venous trunk, the postoperative use of anti-coagulants should be discussed in order to avoid thrombosis of the vascular assemblies [23].

  o *Arterial structures of the mediastinum*: In the case of resections extended to the arterial trunks including the thoracic aorta [24,25], whether limited to the arterial adventitia or to the complete wall with prosthetic replacement, the surgical procedure is most often carried out with circulatory assistance or extracorporeal circulation [26] (CEC), even though it is sometimes not used with good postoperative results [27].

- Cardiac chambers: including the right atrium which represents the most resected cardiac structure [27], most often in association with resection of the superior vena cava [26,28] with reconstructions using pericardial or prosthetic patches.

A more extensive resection associating two or more of these overlying structures is possible (Figure 3), with the final result of ensuring the most carcinological resection possible in a healthy area, while respecting the continuity of the vascular axes and adequate cardiorespiratory function. A complex resection may involve resection of the thymus, superior vena cava, right atrium and lung [29], thymus resection associated with resection of the aortic arch with pneumonectomy [25], or thymus resection associated with mediastinal venous reconstruction and coronary bypass surgery [18].

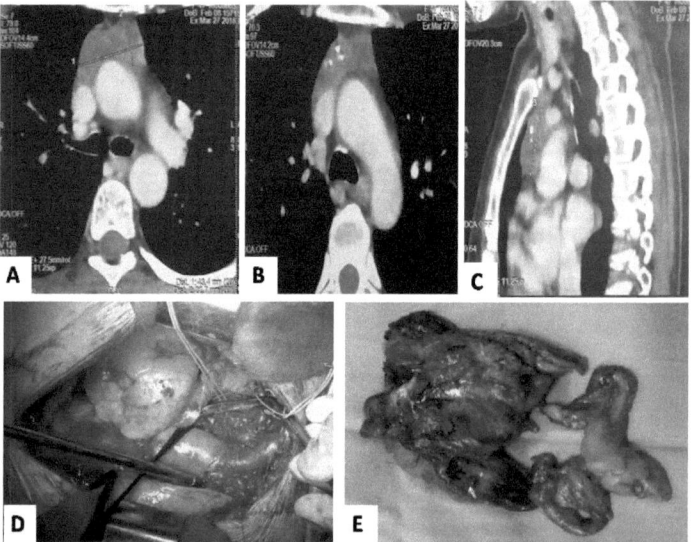

Figure 3 : Invasive thymoma after neo-adjuvant chemotherapy (A,B,C): single-block resection of the thymus enlarged to the inominate venous trunk, the lateral aspect of the superior vena cava, and the pericardium by median sternotomy (D) Surgical specimen (E)

IV- Results of surgery for advanced thymoma :

Surgery for invasive thymoma is correlated with a morbidity of between 15 and 70% and an early mortality within the first three months postoperatively of between 0 and 8%.

A great variability of results is observed according to the surgical teams, the types and extent of resection performed, the histological stages of the resected tumors, the procedure performed and the invaded structures removed with the tumor.

The published series on extended thymic resection and their results are summarized in the following table:

Author	Year	Number	Approach / Gestures	Morbidity	mortality	Survival
Marukawa[14]	2015	13	Nodular resection (11/13) Extra pleural pneumonectomy (2/13)	69.2% recurrences ++.	7.6%	92.3% (5 years)
Sun[30][	2017	25	Vascular resection (VCS or TVI) or OD (100%) Wedge (6) Lobectomy (7) Pericardial resection (19) Pleurectomy (10)	R0 resection (80%) Complications: 52%. of which 32%: postoperative transfusion	8% (3 months)	59.1% (5 years)

Sugiura[12]	1999	40	Complete extended thymic resection (27/40)	Incomplete resection (4/40) Unresectable tumor (9/40).		Stage II: 72% (10 years) Stage III: 47% (10 years) Stage IV: 0%.
Huang[3131]	1997	44	77% invasive thymoma 23% thymic carcinoma	18% of incomplete resections		
Yagi[5]	1996	41	Stage III (34), Stage IVa (5), Stage IVb (2) With Angioplasty or venous reconstruction (12/41)	Occlusion of venous reconstruction (16%)	0%	Stage III: 82% (5 years) Stage IV: 67% (5 years)
Murakawa[32]	2000	140	Stage II (32) Stage III (28) Stage IV (16) Median sternotomy Extended thymectomy	Recurrences (17.8%) of which 84% were stage II or higher.		Overall 84.6% of the total Stage II 96.6 Stage IV 68.4% (5 years)

Post-operative complications vary according to the procedure performed, the surgical approach, and the extent of excision. The need for post-operative transfusions is the most frequent complication in the case of vascular or cardiac reconstructions (of the inominate venous trunk, superior vena cava, thoracic aorta or right atrium). Other possible complications include diaphragmatic paralysis (in case of exeresis extended to the phrenic nerves), pneumopathy and atelectasis (especially after exeresis extended to the lungs), wall infections, and bleeding.

In spite of fairly high morbidity and mortality figures, the quality of surgical excision (essentially R0 type), and the histological stage represent the two essential factors for overall long-term survival. The latter varies between 52 and 92% depending on the series, with better figures observed for stages II compared to stages III and IV.

References:

1. Singh, G., C.M. Rumende, and Z. Amin, *Thymoma: Diagnosis and treatment.* Acta Med Indones, 2011. 43(1): p. 74-8.
2. Liu, C.W., et al, *[Surgical treatment of invasive thymoma: a prognostic retrospective study].* Zhonghua Wai Ke Za Zhi, 2010. 48(12): p. 881-5.

   Schmidt, R., et al, *Surgical therapy of malignant thymoma.* J Cardiovasc Surg (Torino), 1997. 38(3): p. 317-22.
4. Goldman, A.J., et al, *Myasthenia gravis and invasive thymoma: a 20-year experience.* Neurology, 1975. 25(11): p. 1021-5.
5. Yagi, K., et al, *Surgical treatment for invasive thymoma, especially when the superior vena cava is invaded.* Ann Thorac Surg, 1996. 61(2): p. 521-4.
6. Yoshiyasu, N., et al, *Lifesaving surgery for a ruptured invasive thymoma using the hemi-clamshell approach: a case report.* Surg Case Rep, 2019. 5(1): p. 35.
7. Funaki, S., et al, *Surgical treatment strategies for invasive thymoma.* J Thorac Dis, 2020. 12(12): p. 7619-7625.

   Noda, M., et al, *[Video-assisted thoracoscopic surgery of bilateral dissemination of invasive thymoma: report of a case].* Kyobu Geka, 1997. 50(10): p. 886-9.
9. Jiang, J.H., et al, *Modified Subxiphoid Thoracoscopic Thymectomy for Locally Invasive Thymoma.* Ann Thorac Surg, 2020. 27(20): p. 32009-9.
10. Joalsen, I., et al, *Extended thymectomy via subxiphoid uniportal Video-Assisted Thoracoscopic Surgery: A case report.* Int J Surg Case Rep, 2021. 80(105681): p. 105681.
11. Abu-Akar, F., et al. *Subxiphoid Uniportal VATS for Thymic and Combined Mediastinal and Pulmonary Resections - A Two-Year Experience.* Semin Thorac Cardiovasc Surg, 2019. 31(3): p. 614-619.

    Sugiura, H., et al, *Long-term results of surgical treatment for invasive thymoma.* Anticancer Res, 1999. 19(2B): p. 1433-7.

    Kataoka, D., et al, *[Experience with invasive thymoma presenting pleural dissemination].* Kyobu Geka, 2003. 56(12): p. 1025-8.
14. Murakawa, T., et al. *Invasive thymoma disseminated into the pleural cavity: mid-term results of surgical resection.* Eur J Cardiothorac Surg, 2015. 47(3): p. 567-72.

15. Salati, M., et al, *Iatrogenic phrenic nerve injury during thymectomy: the extent of the problem.* J Thorac Cardiovasc Surg, 2010. 139(4): p. e77-8.
16. Grande-Martín, A., et al. *Intraoperative neurophysiological monitoring of the phrenic nerve: utility and descriptions of the technique.* Cir Esp (Engl Ed), 2019. 97(2): p. 103-107.
17. Nomori, H. and H. Horio, *[A case of post-thymomectomy myasthenia gravis after extrapleural pneumonectomy for invasive thymoma which necessitated long-term mechanical ventilation].* Nihon Kokyuki Gakkai Zasshi, 2001. 39(1): p. 66-70.

    Mendez-Fernandez, M.A., et al, *Reconstruction of the left innominate vein in a patient with invasive thymoma undergoing coronary artery bypass surgery.* J Cardiovasc Surg (Torino), 1986. 27(3): p. 351-4.
19. Kumar, A., et al, *Superior Vena Cava Resection in Locally Advanced Thymoma-Surgical and Survival Outcomes.* Indian J Surg Oncol, 2020. 11(4): p. 711-719.
20. Galbis Caravajal, J., et al, *[Extensive surgical resection in the treatment of invasive thymoma].* Clin Transl Oncol, 2005. 7(3): p. 130-2.
21. Sakamaki, Y., H. Shiono, and T. Miura, *[Invasive thymoma with extensive growth in the superior vena cava;report of a case].* Kyobu Geka, 2012. 65(10): p. 926-9.
22. Umeda, Y., et al, *[Reconstruction of the superior vena cava for invasive thymoma under monitoring of regional cerebral saturation of oxygen].* Kyobu Geka, 2014. 67(10): p. 873-6.
23. Arvind, K., et al, *Resection and reconstruction of mediastinal great vessels in invasive thymoma.* Indian J Cancer, 2010. 47(4): p. 400-5.
24. Fujino, S., et al, *Reconstruction of the aortic arch in invasive thymoma under retrograde cerebral perfusion.* Ann Thorac Surg, 1998. 66(1): p. 263-4.
25. Ayabe, T., et al, *[Complete resection of the invasive thymoma combined with replacement of aortic arch and pneumonectomy].* Kyobu Geka, 2006. 59(9): p. 804-8.
26. Dong, Y.Q., et al. *Surgical treatment of an invasive thymoma extending into the superior vena cava and right atrium.* World J Surg Oncol, 2014. 12(6): p. 6.
27. Gleeson, R.E., et al. *invasive thymoma extending to the right atrium: excision without cardiopulmonary bypass.* J Cardiovasc Surg (Torino), 1997. 38(4): p. 429-31.

28. Li, W., et al, *Resection of an invasive thymoma extending into the superior vena cava and right atrium.* J Card Surg, 2010. 25(5): p. 515-7.
29. Shudo, Y., et al, *Radical operation for invasive thymoma with intracaval, intracardiac, and lung invasion.* J Card Surg, 2007. 22(4): p. 330-2.
30. Sun, Y., et al. *Reconstruction of mediastinal vessels for invasive thymoma: a retrospective analysis of 25 cases.* J Thorac Dis, 2017. 9(3): p. 725-733.
31. Huang, H.Y. and W.J. Chen, *Malignant thymoma: a review of 44 cases.* Changgeng Yi Xue Za Zhi, 1997. 20(3): p. 174-80.
    Murakawa, T., et al, *Results from surgical treatment for thymoma. 43 years of experience.* Jpn J Thorac Cardiovasc Surg, 2000. 48(2): p. 89-95.

Place of radiotherapy in the treatment of epithelial tumors of the thymus

Fatma Elloumi1,3, Mariem Frikha1,3, Ines Ayadi2,3, Jamel Daoud1,3
(1) Department of carcinological radiotherapy CHU Habib Bourguiba Sfax
(2) Medical carcinology department CHU Hbib Bourguiba Sfax
(3) Faculty of Medicine of Sfax Tunisia

Summary:

At present, surgical resection is the cornerstone of treatment for resectable thymic tumors. Postoperative radiotherapy is indicated in cases of incomplete resection, invasive (stage III) and histologically aggressive tumours (B3 thymoma or thymic carcinoma).

For unresectable thymic tumours, the therapeutic strategy is multimodal and is based on chemotherapy followed by local treatment by surgery or radiotherapy.

In the presence of distant metastases, systemic therapies are the main recourse to improve the quality of life of these patients.

The prognostic factors for TETs are mainly represented by the stage of the disease, the histological type and the completeness of the resection

I- Introduction:

Thymic epithelial tumors (TETs) are a heterogeneous group that includes thymomas and thymic carcinomas. They belong to the group of orphan tumors [1].

These tumors represent 20% of all mediastinal tumors and nearly 50% of tumor processes in the anterior mediastinum [2]. They often develop within the thymic cavity but can have ectopic topographies, particularly in the cervical-mediastinum region [2].

The disease is often revealed by a para-thymic syndrome related to an autoimmune disorder, the most common of which is myasthenia gravis [3].

Signs of compression or locoregional invasion may reveal TETs [3].

The thoracic CT scan is the reference examination in the pre-therapeutic assessment [4].

Currently, surgery remains the cornerstone of treatment for resectable thymic epithelial tumors [5]. 5] Decisions on adjuvant treatment with postoperative radiotherapy and/or adjuvant chemotherapy are complex and must take into account histological type, quality of excision, and tumor stage [4].

Locally advanced TETs considered unresectable should benefit from multimodal treatment including induction chemotherapy followed by surgical resection or radiotherapy depending on response [4].

We propose to document the role of radiotherapy in the therapeutic management of TET.

II- Post-operative Radiotherapy:

Due to the lack of large enough prospective studies and randomized trials, there is no consensus on the indications and modalities of postoperative radiotherapy. They depend mainly on three criteria:

- ❖ The quality of the resection
- ❖ Masaoka-Koga Stadium
- ❖ The histopathological subtype

Until the 1980s, adjuvant radiotherapy was performed in all patients operated on for a thymic tumor, regardless of the stage or quality of resection. This attitude has been challenged by more recent work [6].

Zhang et al had demonstrated in a prospective randomized study of 29 patients treated for Masaoka-Koga stage I TET the lack of benefit of adjuvant radiotherapy. The overall survival at 10 years was 88% for the adjuvant radiotherapy arm versus 92% for the surgery alone arm with ($P > 0.05$) [7].

The results of the American SEER (Surveillance, Epidemiology, and End Results program) on data from 901 patients showed no survival benefit for stage I. These same results were in favour of adjuvant radiotherapy for stages II and III with an overall survival at 5 years of 76% for patients treated with adjuvant radiotherapy compared to 66% for patients treated with surgery alone (p =0.01).

In subgroup analysis, the benefit of adjuvant radiotherapy was found only in patients with incomplete resection (R1 or R2). Adjuvant radiotherapy for stage II and III patients with complete resection had no benefit in terms of progression-free survival or overall survival [8].

An analysis of retrospective data from 13 studies corroborates these findings in 592 patients with stage II and III TET after R0 surgery. The risk of recurrence was similar in the groups with and without radiotherapy [9].

In 2016, in a retrospective study conducted by ITMIG including 1263 patients, treated for Masoaka -koga stage II -III TET with R0 resection, 5-year overall survival was 95% with post -operative radiotherapy versus 86% without radiotherapy (p=0.002).

In subgroup analysis, the gain was more significant in stage III and in subtypes B1, B2 and B3 [10].

The indications for adjuvant radiotherapy according to the latest RYTHMIC 2020 guideline were defined according to the quality of resection (R0 or R1/R2), Masaoka-Koga stage, and histological type [11].

In case of complete resection, radiotherapy is not indicated in patients with Masaoka-Koga stage I, stage IIA type A to B2 and stage IIB type A to B1 disease [11].

On the other hand, postoperative radiotherapy is indicated in patients with stage IIA and type B3 thymic tumor, stage IIB and type B2 or B3, stages III and IV regardless of type [12, 13].

If resection is incomplete (R1/R2), radiation therapy is indicated regardless of stage and histological type [11].

After complete resection of thymic carcinoma, postoperative radiotherapy is an option for stage I tumors, should be offered for stage II tumors, and is recommended for stage III / IVA tumors [7,14].

III- Neoadjuvant radiotherapy:

There are no randomized studies examining the place and value of neoadjuvant radiotherapy. In a phase II trial, Robert J et al evaluated the value of a combination of chemotherapy and preoperative radiotherapy for inoperable tumors. The study included 22 patients treated with two courses of platinum-based chemotherapy and etoposide followed by radiotherapy at a dose of 45 Gy. The primary objective of the study was the objective response rate. The secondary objectives were toxicity and complete resection. Seventeen patients underwent surgery with R0 resection. Five of the patients had less than 10% viable tumor. The toxicity was also acceptable[15].

In another retrospective study by Cameron including 10 patients with locally advanced stage III and IV NET treated with 2 courses of cisplatin and Etoposide chemotherapy concomitantly with radiotherapy (40-45Gy), the complete response rate with R0 resection was 80% and the overall survival at 5 years was 69% with acceptable toxicity [16].

A review of the literature was published in 2017 by Michial including 3 retrospective studies. The author concluded that the combination of chemotherapy and preoperative radiotherapy increases the rate of complete resection with increased toxicity and more difficult surgery given the presence of fibrosis [17].

IV- Exclusive radiotherapy :

Radiotherapy is proposed as an alternative to surgery in cases of unresectable tumours or in cases where surgery is medically contraindicated. In this case, radiotherapy is often combined with chemotherapy.

Phase II trials have shown that response rates in stage IV patients treated with radiotherapy and chemotherapy range from 40% to 60% in thymoma and from 20% to 40% in thymic carcinoma. Progression-free survival after exclusive radiotherapy was 9 to 26 months for thymoma and 5 to 7 months for thymic carcinoma[18,19].

In a retrospective study by Jumpei et al in 2017, about 20 patients with thymoma or stage IVA/IVB thymic carcinoma treated with radiotherapy and chemotherapy, response rates ranged from 57% to 67%. Progression-free survival was 15 months for thymic carcinoma and 38 months for thymoma with 5-year survival rates of 63% for thymoma and 26% for thymic carcinoma [20].

For chemotherapy protocols, given the small number of patients, there are no randomized controlled trials in the literature comparing different chemotherapy protocols.

The CAP Cisplatin (50 mg/m2), Adriamycin (50 mg/m2), Cyclophosphamide (500 mg/m2) protocol administered every 21 days is the most commonly used protocol and probably gives the best response rates between 50% and 70% [21].

Loehrer evaluated the CAP protocol in 30 metastatic and recurrent patients (54% had radiotherapy). The objective response rate obtained was 50% with a median survival of 12 months [21].

In a phase II trial conducted by KIMES evaluating the place of the CAP protocol as neoadjuvant before surgery, including 22 patients (50% stage III, 50% stage IV), all patients had postoperative radiotherapy with an objective response rate at CT of 80% and an overall survival rate at 5 years of 95% [22].

Combinations of carboplatin (AUC 5 to 6) and paclitaxel (150 to 200 mg/m2), ADOC (Cisplatin (50 mg/m2), Adriamycin (50 mg/m2), Vincristine (0.6 mg/m2) and Cyclophosphamide (700 mg/m2) or VIP (Etoposide 75mg/m2, Ifosfamide1.8g/m2 and Cisplatin20mg/m2) every 21 days are the most commonly used combinations after CAP[18, 23].

According to data from an EORTC [European Organization On Research And Treatment Of Cancer] study testing the VIP protocol in combination with radiotherapy, the objective response rate was 60%. Thirty percent of patients (30%) were in complete remission with a median survival of 4.3 years. Loehrer reported an objective response rate of 43% with VIP in metastatic and/or recurrent patients [24].

The different chemotherapy protocols are summarized in the following table [25].

Author	Number	Type	Method	Protocol	Response rate
Fornasiero et al. 1990	32 [26]	Thymoma	Retrospective	ADOC	85-92 %
Loehrer et al. 1994	30[27]	Thymoma and thymic carcinoma	Phase II	CAP	51 %
Giaccone et al. 1996	16 [28]	Thymoma	Phase II	PE	56-60%
Loehrer et al. 2001	34 [29]	Thymoma and thymic carcinoma	Phase II	VIP	32%
Lemma et al. 2008	46 [30]	Thymoma and thymic carcinoma	Phase II	Carbo-Paclitaxel	33%

V- Palliative radiotherapy :

Radiotherapy may be indicated in the palliative situation:

- decompressive: in case of superior cave syndrome. [31]

Superior vena cava compression syndrome may be secondary to infiltrating thymic tumors. It is an emergency that may be due to either direct tumor invasion or external compression or thrombosis. Symptoms include swelling of the face, neck, arms and chest, difficulty breathing, headache and dizziness.

Thymic carcinoma is responsible for 3.4% of the aetiologies of upper cava syndromes [32].

- radiotherapy of bone metastases: the aim is usually analgesic. It also prolongs the patient's ambulatory state and reduces the risk of fractures and compression.

VI- Conclusion:

The value of adjuvant radiotherapy has been demonstrated for TETs in cases of incomplete resection. In the case of complete surgery, the indication for radiation therapy takes into account the histological grade.

Radiotherapy is an alternative to surgery for unresectable infiltrating tumours. The combination of chemotherapy is recommended for locally advanced forms.

References:

[1] Robinson SP, Akhondi H. Thymoma. StatPearls, Treasure Island (FL): StatPearls Publishing; 2021.

[2] Engels EA, Pfeiffer RM. Malignant thymoma in the United States: demographic patterns in incidence and associations with subsequent malignancies. Int J Cancer 2003;105:546-51.

[3] Rosenow EC, Hurley BT. Disorders of the thymus. A review. Arch Intern Med 1984;144:763-70.

[4] Girard N, Ruffini E, Marx A, Faivre-Finn C, Peters S, ESMO Guidelines Committee. Thymic epithelial tumours: ESMO Clinical Practice Guidelines for diagnosis, treatment and follow-up. Ann Oncol Off J Eur Soc Med Oncol 2015;26 Suppl 5:v 40-55.

[5] Falkson CB, Bezjak A, Darling G, Gregg R, Malthaner R, Maziak DE, et al. The management of thymoma: a systematic review and practice

guideline. J Thorac Oncol Off Publ Int Assoc Study Lung Cancer 2009;4:911-9.

[6] document.pdf n.d.

[7] Zhang H, Lu N, Wang M, Gu X, Zhang D. Postoperative radiotherapy for stage I thymoma: a prospective randomized trial in 29 cases. Chin Med J (Engl) 1999;112:136-8.

[8] Forquer JA, Rong N, Fakiris AJ, Loehrer PJ, Johnstone PAS. Postoperative radiotherapy after surgical resection of thymoma: differing roles in localized and regional disease. Int J Radiat Oncol Biol Phys 2010;76:440-5.

[9] Korst RJ, Kansler AL, Christos PJ, Mandal S. Adjuvant radiotherapy for thymic epithelial tumors: a systematic review and meta-analysis. Ann Thorac Surg 2009;87:1641-7.

[10] Rimner A, Yao X, Huang J, Antonicelli A, Ahmad U, Korst RJ, et al. Postoperative Radiation Therapy Is Associated with Longer Overall Survival in Completely Resected Stage II and III Thymoma-An Analysis of the International Thymic Malignancies Interest Group Retrospective Database. J Thorac Oncol Off Publ Int Assoc Study Lung Cancer 2016;11:1785-92.

[11] referentiel_RYTHMIC_2020.pdf n.a.

[12] Gao L, Wang C, Fang W, Zhang J, Lv C, Fu S. Outcome of multimodality treatment for 188 cases of type B3 thymoma. J Thorac Oncol Off Publ Int Assoc Study Lung Cancer 2013;8:1329-34.

[13] Weksler B, Shende M, Nason KS, Gallagher A, Ferson PF, Pennathur A. The role of adjuvant radiation therapy for resected stage III thymoma: a population-based study. Ann Thorac Surg 2012;93:1822-8; discussion 1828-1829.

[14] Ruffini E, Detterbeck F, Van Raemdonck D, Rocco G, Thomas P, Weder W, et al. Thymic carcinoma: a cohort study of patients from the European

society of thoracic surgeons database. J Thorac Oncol Off Publ Int Assoc Study Lung Cancer 2014;9:541-8.

[15] Korst RJ, Bezjak A, Blackmon S, Choi N, Fidias P, Liu G, et al. Neoadjuvant chemoradiotherapy for locally advanced thymic tumors: a phase II, multi-institutional clinical trial. J Thorac Cardiovasc Surg 2014;147:36-44, 46.e1.

[16] Wright CD, Choi NC, Wain JC, Mathisen DJ, Lynch TJ, Fidias P. Induction chemoradiotherapy followed by resection for locally advanced Masaoka stage III and IVA thymic tumors. Ann Thorac Surg 2008;85:385-9.

[17] Lanuti M. Induction chemoradiotherapy for unresectable thymic tumors. Mediastinum 2017;1.

[18] Hirai F, Yamanaka T, Taguchi K, Daga H, Ono A, Tanaka K, et al. A multicenter phase II study of carboplatin and paclitaxel for advanced thymic carcinoma: WJOG4207L. Ann Oncol Off J Eur Soc Med Oncol 2015;26:363-8.

[19] Kunitoh H, Tamura T, Shibata T, Nakagawa K, Takeda K, Nishiwaki Y, et al. A phase-II trial of dose-dense chemotherapy in patients with disseminated thymoma: report of a Japan Clinical Oncology Group trial (JCOG 9605). Br J Cancer 2009;101:1549-54.

[20] Kashima J, Okuma Y, Murata H, Watanabe K, Hosomi Y, Hishima T. Chemoradiotherapy for unresectable cases of thymic epithelial tumors: a retrospective study. J Thorac Dis 2017;9:3911-8.

[21] Grassin F, Paleiron N, André M, Caliandro R, Bretel J-J, Terrier P, et al. Combined Etoposide, Ifosfamide, and Cisplatin in the Treatment of Patients with Advanced Thymoma and Thymic Carcinoma. A French Experience. J Thorac Oncol 2010;5:893-7.

[22] Kim ES, Putnam JB, Komaki R, Walsh GL, Ro JY, Shin HJ, et al. Phase II study of a multidisciplinary approach with induction

chemotherapy, followed by surgical resection, radiation therapy, and consolidation chemotherapy for unresectable malignant thymomas: final report. Lung Cancer Amst Neth 2004;44:369-79.

[23] Lemma GL, Lee J-W, Aisner SC, Langer CJ, Tester WJ, Johnson DH, et al. Phase II study of carboplatin and paclitaxel in advanced thymoma and thymic carcinoma. J Clin Oncol Off J Am Soc Clin Oncol 2011;29:2060-5.

[24] Gomez D, Komaki R, Yu J, Ikushima H, Bezjak A. Radiation therapy definitions and reporting guidelines for thymic malignancies. J Thorac Oncol Off Publ Int Assoc Study Lung Cancer 2011;6:S1743-1748.

[25] Girard N, Lal R, Wakelee H, Riely GJ, Loehrer PJ. Chemotherapy definitions and policies for thymic malignancies. J Thorac Oncol Off Publ Int Assoc Study Lung Cancer 2011;6:S1749-1755.

[26] Arbib et al - 2016 - RYTHMIC network), F. BARLESI, J. BENNOUNA, L. CHALA.pdf n.d.

[27] Dahan M, Gaillard J, Mary H, Renella-Coll J, Berjaud J. [Long-term survival of surgically treated lympho-epithelial thymomas]. Rev Mal Respir 1988;5:159-65.

[28] Huang J, Rizk NP, Travis WD, Riely GJ, Park BJ, Bains MS, et al. Comparison of patterns of relapse in thymic carcinoma and thymoma. J Thorac Cardiovasc Surg 2009;138:26-31.

[29] Detterbeck FC, Parsons AM. Thymic tumors. Ann Thorac Surg 2004;77:1860-9.

[30] Blumberg D, Port JL, Weksler B, Delgado R, Rosai J, Bains MS, et al. Thymoma: a multivariate analysis of factors predicting survival. Ann Thorac Surg 1995;60:908-13; discussion 914.

[31] Lalani N, Brade AM. Radiation dose for thymic tumours. Mediastinum 2020;4.

[32] Berny M, Zaghba N, Benjelloune H, Yassine N. Etiological profile of superior cave syndrome. Rev Mal Respir 2016;33:A94.

[33] Gomez D, Komaki R, Yu J, Ikushima H, Bezjak A. Radiation therapy definitions and reporting guidelines for thymic malignancies. J Thorac Oncol Off Publ Int Assoc Study Lung Cancer 2011;6:S1743-1748.

Radiotherapy of TET: Technical aspects and side effects

Fatma Elloumi[1,2], Mariem Frikha[1,2], Jamel Daoud[1,2]

(1) Department of carcinological radiotherapy CHU Habib Bourguiba Sfax
(2) Faculty of Medicine of Sfax Tunisia

I- Introduction:

Current practice for mediastinal radiotherapy of TETs varies widely in terms of target volume definition. Recommended doses depend on the status of the margins.

In this article, we propose to clarify the technical aspects of this irradiation and the side effects that result from it.

II- Contouring of target volumes:

The target volumes are outlined on a thoracic scanner in the treatment position with a 3 mm slice pitch. An injection of contrast medium is recommended in the absence of contraindications.

Recommendations for contouring target volumes are based on expert agreement [1, 2].

- **GTV** : (Gross Tumor Volume): corresponds to the macroscopic tumor visible on CT or MRI or PET scan in case of unresectable tumor and to the tumor residue in case of incomplete resection.

CTV : (Clinical Target Volume):

For unresectable tumors, it includes the GTV, as well as subclinical extensions not visible on imaging. The CTV is defined by the GTV with margins of 0.5 to 1 cm according to the experts [1].

Postoperatively, this volume corresponds to the tumour bed. The target volume includes the entire thymic cavity and any tumour extensions (pericardium, large vessels, pleura, pulmonary parenchyma, etc.). The radiopaque clips placed intraoperatively at the level of the tumour bed, areas of adhesions or in case of doubt about a marginal limit, are of great help in defining this volume.

The contouring is done according to the clinical data, the imaging, the surgical report, the anatomopathological report, taking into account the natural history of the disease.

- **PTV** (planning Target volume): is defined by the CTV and a safety margin that allows for positioning uncertainties, possible organ and patient movements, and dose homogeneity problems within the target volume.

PTV recommended by experts = CTV + 0.5 to 1.5 cm margins [1].

III . Dose of radiation therapy:

Postoperatively, the radiation doses for thymic tumors are much debated. After complete R0 resection, the recommended dose is between 45 and 56 Gy in the whole target volume, in standard fractionation (1.8 to 2 Gy per session) [3].

In case of R1 resection, additional radiation up to 66 Gy is delivered to the area where resection would be insufficient. The use of surgical clips allows the precise definition of areas of insufficient or doubtful resection [3].

In the case of unresectable tumors or residual tumors, the recommended dose is 66 Gy [2]. Radiation therapy is often combined with chemotherapy sequentially or concomitantly [4-6].

According to the RYTHMIC guidelines, adjuvant radiotherapy should be started within 3 months after surgery [2].

IV. Organ at Risk (OAR) and Dose Constraints:

Dose constraints to healthy tissues are those for external thoracic radiotherapy [4]. Recommendations published by Gomez et al, have been approved by ITGM members regarding dose constraints [4] :

- Spinal cord: the maximum dose is 45 Gy in conventional fractionation
- Healthy lung - PTV: a dose of 20 Gy should not be delivered in more than 35% of the volume and a dose of 30 Gy should not be exceeded in more than 20% of the lung volume.

    The recommended average dose should be less than 13 Gy according to EMAMI dose constraints and 20 Gy according to RTOG dose constraints [7-9].

- Heart: the 30 Gy dose should not be delivered to more than 46% of the volume (QUANTEC/EMAMI) [7, 9].

    The dose of 35 Gy should not be delivered to more than 30% of the volume (SFRO) [10].

    The maximum dose is 35 Gy throughout the heart. A maximum limitation of the cardiac volume receiving 40 Gy is mandatory. The recommended average dose is 26 Gy.

- Esophagus: the maximum recommended dose is 40 Gy over a length of 15 cm.

    According to EMAMI, the maximum dose to the esophagus can be up to 74 Gy.

    The average dose should not exceed 34 Gy according to SFRO and RTOG recommendations [8, 10].

Table I summarizes the dosimetric constraints based on recommendations published by Gomez et al and approved by ITGM members [1].

Organs	RT only	RT combined with CT
Healthy lung -PTV	Dmoy < 20 Gy V20 <40%	Dmoy < 20 Gy V20 < 35% V10 < 45% V5 < 65%
Heart	V30 < 45% Dmoy < 26 Gy	V30 <45% Dmoy < 26 Gy
Spinal cord	Dmax<45 Gy	Dmax < 45Gy
Esophagus	Dmax < 80 Gy Dmoy < 34 Gy V70 < 20% V50 < 50%	Dmax < 80Gy Dmoy < 34Gy V70 < 20% V50 < 40%

V. Radiotherapy Techniques

Previously, RT of TETs was delivered with conventional techniques using orthogonal beams with successive reductions to preserve organs at risk, particularly the spinal cord [11].

Nevertheless, given the progress made in radiation technology in recent years, several other techniques are possible.

- Three-dimensional conformal radiotherapy (3D-CRT) is the most widely used technique. It allows the shape of the radiation beam to be matched as closely as possible to the volume to be treated (Figure A).

- Intensity modulated conformal radiotherapy (IMRT): The variation of the beam intensity along the surface to be irradiated offers very complex dose distributions, shaped around the different volumes to be irradiated and preserving the volumes to be spared (Figure B). This technique also allows dose escalation to target volumes with reduced toxicity especially in the heart [12]

Although there is no direct comparison between 3D RT and IMRT in the setting of TET, IMRT has proven to be superior in several studies with respect to compliance with doses to organs at risk [1]

- Proton therapy: Thanks to the physical characteristics of protons, the dose is limited in the non-tumourous zones crossed. It is maximal at the level of the cancerous target and almost zero beyond [13]. According to Catherine E, in a prospective study published in 2018, conducted between 2008 and 2017, including 30 patients with TET treated with proton therapy, this technique guarantees a good local control with a suitable toxicity profile [14].

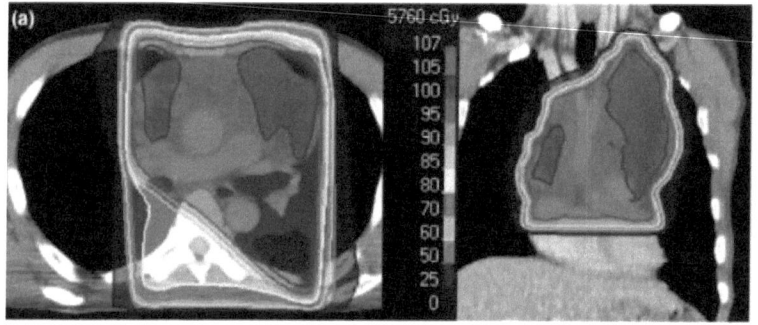

Figure A: Dose distribution using 3D conformal RT

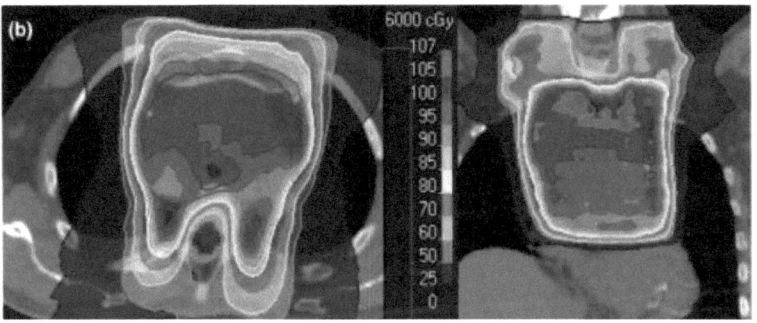

Figure 1: Dose Distribution by IMRT Technique

VII. Side effects of radiotherapy :

Acute toxicity :

- **Cutaneous toxicity:** radiodermatitis is manifested by progressive cutaneous erythema from 10 to 20Gy, oedema of the cutaneous and subcutaneous tissues, dry and then exudative desquamation, and even cutaneous ulceration, which may lead in rare cases to cutaneous necrosis.

- **Acute esophagitis and fungal superinfection:** clinical symptoms are dominated by dysphagia and odynophagia, sometimes requiring enteral or parenteral nutrition.

- **Acute pericarditis** suspected in the presence of chest pain, fever and sometimes ST segment abnormalities on the electrocardiogram.

- **Acute lung disease**: most often manifested by dyspnea with dry cough

- **Dyspnea: from** a simple shortness of breath during a moderate effort to dyspnea at rest

- **General reactions:** asthenia or fatigue, loss of appetite, weight loss, nausea, vomiting.

The scoring of the various acute side effects is done according to the RTOG scale (see Appendix I) or according to the National Cancer Institute (NCI) Common Terminology Criteria for Adverse Events (CTC AE) version 4 (see Appendix II).

According to a recently published Italian retrospective study, which included 183 patients, 114 of whom underwent postoperative radiotherapy, 39.5% of the patients presented an acute toxicity of Grade < III according to the CTC AE version 4 scale. The rates of acute pulmonary toxicity, esophagitis and acute cardiac toxicity were 8%, 34.2%, 0.9% respectively [13].

2- Late toxicity:

Late complications are rare and involve:

- The skin: of the cutaneous fibrosis type.
- Lung parenchyma: pulmonary fibrosis.
- Pericardium: Late exudative pericarditis.
- Spinal cord: Radiation myelitis.
- Esophagus: Late stenosis, rarely perforation.

According to the same study by Bruni, the rate of late toxicity was 20% and patients who developed acute toxicities had a higher risk of developing late toxicity [15]

In a study conducted by Liao, the objective was to evaluate the relationship between the average cardiac dose and the risk of cardiovascular disease. This study included 130 patients with stage III thymoma (74 patients treated with surgery + postoperative RT, 31 patients had exclusive radiotherapy). The author concluded that the mean cardiac dose was an independent factor of cardiovascular disease [16].

According to Vitali et al, in a retrospective study that collated 55 patients treated with radiotherapy for TETs, the mean lung dose was strongly correlated with late pulmonary complications and the risk of fibrosis with a mean lung dose Cut off of 20 Gy [17].

VIII- Conclusion :

The correct definition of target volumes is essential for the success of postoperative TET irradiation. The contouring of these volumes must take into account all the elements of the file: radiological, intraoperative and anatomopathological.

New radiotherapy techniques, particularly intensity modulated radiotherapy, ensure adequate coverage of target volumes while respecting dose constraints for organs at risk.

References:

[1] Gomez D, Komaki R, Yu J, Ikushima H, Bezjak A. Radiation therapy definitions and reporting guidelines for thymic malignancies. J Thorac Oncol Off Publ Int Assoc Study Lung Cancer 2011;6:S1743-1748.

[2] referentiel_RYTHMIC_2020.pdf

[3] Lalani N, Brade AM. Radiation dose for thymic tumours. Mediastinum 2020;4.

[4] Maggi L, Andreetta F, Antozzi C, Baggi F, Bernasconi P, Cavalcante P, et al. Thymoma-associated myasthenia gravis: outcome, clinical and pathological correlations in 197 patients on a 20-year experience. J Neuroimmunol 2008;201-202:237-44.

[5] Girard N, Mornex F. The role of radiotherapy in the management of thymic tumors. Thorac Surg Clin 2011;21:99-105, vii.

[6] Mornex F, Resbeut M, Richaud P, Jung GM, Mirabel X, Marchal C, et al. Radiotherapy and chemotherapy for invasive thymomas: a multicentric retrospective review of 90 cases. The FNCLCC trialists. Fédération Nationale des Centres de Lutte Contre le Cancer. Int J Radiat Oncol Biol Phys 1995;32:651-9.

[7] Emami B, Lyman J, Brown A, Coia L, Goitein M, Munzenrider JE, et al. Tolerance of normal tissue to therapeutic irradiation. Int J Radiat Oncol Biol Phys 1991;21:109-22.

[8] Radiation Oncology/Toxicity/RTOG - Wikibooks, open books for an open world n.d.

[9] Rep_Radiother_Oncol_2013_1_1_35_48.

[10] Noël G, Antoni D, Barillot I, Chauvet B. Delineation of organs at risk and dosimetric constraints. Cancer/Radiotherapy 2016;20:S36-60.

[11] Gomez D, Komaki R. Technical advances of radiation therapy for thymic malignancies. J Thorac Oncol Off Publ Int Assoc Study Lung Cancer 2010;5:S336-343.

[12] Franceschini D, Cozzi L, Loi M, Franzese C, Reggiori G, Mancosu P, et al. Volumetric modulated arc therapy versus intensity-modulated proton therapy in the postoperative irradiation of thymoma. J Cancer Res Clin Oncol 2020;146:2267-76.

[13] Willmann J, Rimner A. The expanding role of radiation therapy for thymic malignancies. J Thorac Dis 2018;10:S2555-64.

[14] Mercado CE, Hartsell WF, Simone CB, Tsai HK, Vargas CE, Zhu HJ, et al. Proton therapy for thymic malignancies: multi-institutional patterns-of-care and early clinical outcomes from the proton collaborative group and the university of Florida prospective registries. Acta Oncol Stockh Swed 2019;58:1036-40.

[15] Bruni A, Stefani A, Perna M, Borghetti P, Giaj Levra N, D'Angelo E, et al. The role of postoperative radiotherapy for thymomas: a multicentric retrospective evaluation from three Italian centers and review of the literature. J Thorac Dis 2020;12:7518-30.

[16] Liao J, Liu T, Zhang H, Cai F, Chen J, Dang J. The role of postoperative radiation therapy for completely resected stage III thymoma and effect of higher heart radiation dose on risk of cardiovascular disease: A retrospective cohort study. Int J Surg Lond Engl 2018;53:345-9.

[17] Robinson SP, Akhondi H. Thymoma. StatPearls, Treasure Island (FL): StatPearls Publishing; 2021.

Appendix I: RTOG Dermal Toxicity Scoring

Toxicité cutanée (RTOG) :

- **Grade 0 :** Pas de modification par rapport à l'état initial
- **Grade 1 :** Folliculaires, érythème pâle ou terne/ épilation / desquamation sèche / diminution de la transpiration
- **Grade 2 :** Érythème tendre ou lumineux, desquamation humide incomplète/ œdème modéré
- **Grade 3 :** Desquamation humide confluente autre que les plis cutanés, œdème
- **Grade 4 :** Ulcération / Hémorragie / Nécrose
- **Grade 5 :** Décès

Appendix II: Acute Toxicity Scores from the CTC AE Version 4 Scale

	Skin Dermatitis	*Esophagitis*	*Dyspnea*	*Dysphagia*	*Pulmonary fibrosis*
Grade I	Faint erythema or scaling dryer	Asymptomatic; diagnosis at clinical examination only; no treatment required	Shortness of breath during moderate effort	Symptomatic, normal diet	Mild hypoxemia; X-ray pulmonary fibrosis <25% of lung volume
Grade II	Moderate to severe erythema; scaling oozing in patches, mainly affecting the skin folds and creases; moderate edema	Symptomatic; disorders for eating / swallowing; requiring a oral supplementation	Shortness of breath with minimal effort interfering with instrumental activities of daily living	Symptomatic and eating/swallowing disorders	Severe hypoxemia; signs right heart failure; X-ray pulmonary fibrosis > 50 - 75
Grade III	Oozing plaque desquamation, affecting areas other than skin folds and creases; bleeding induced by minor trauma or abrasions	Severe eating disorders / swallowing; requiring a feeding tube enteral nutrition, total parenteral nutrition or hospitalization	Shortness of breath at rest; interfering with the basic activities of life daily	Severe eating disorders / swallowing; requiring a feeding tube enteral nutrition or total parenteral nutrition or a hospitalization	Moderate hypoxemia; signs of pulmonary hypertension; pulmonary fibrosis on X-ray 25 - 50
Grade IV	Life-threatening ; skin necrosis or full-thickness ulceration of the dermis; spontaneous bleeding from affected sites; indication for skin grafting	Life-threatening ; emergency surgery required	Life-threatening requiring emergency treatment	Life-threatening requiring emergency treatment	Life-threatening (eg: hemodynamic, pulmonary complications) requiring intubation with ventilatory assistance; X-ray pulmonary fibrosis > 75% with major honeycomb appearance
Grade V	Deaths	Deaths	Deaths	Deaths	Deaths

Systemic treatment of thymic epithelial tumors

Ines AYADI[1,2], Fatma Elloumi[1,3], Afef KHANFIR[1,2]

1-Faculty of Medicine of Sfax

2-Medical oncology department, CHU Habib Bourguiba Sfax

3-Service of carcinological radiotherapy CHU Hbib Bourguiba Sfax

Tunisia

Summary:

Thymic epithelial tumours (TETs) are rare tumours for which surgery is the cornerstone of treatment. Adjuvant systemic therapy is usually not offered in this setting. However, in locally advanced, unresectable TET, induction chemotherapy (CT) with cisplatin is standard for secondary locoregional treatment. In metastatic or relapsed TET, cisplatin-based CT should be offered as first-line therapy. In second line, several therapeutic weapons can be used, i.e. 2nd line CT or targeted therapy with antiangiogenic drugs (Sunitinib or Levatinib), m-TOR inhibitor (Everolimus) or Octreotide after a positive octreotide scan. Immunotherapy with pembrolizumab can also be proposed as a second line treatment for thymic carcinoma after a prior autoimmune workup.

I. Introduction:

The management of Thymic Epithelial Tumors (TETs) is multidisciplinary. Surgery is the cornerstone of treatment for resectable TEK. Radiation therapy (RT) is usually discussed in cases of non-resectability or non-carcinological limitations. Systemic chemotherapy (CT) is discussed for metastatic, unresectable or relapsed TETs [1]. Targeted therapies and immunotherapy have been shown to be effective in the management of refractory TETs [2].

II. Chemotherapy:

The role of CT in the management of TETs is discussed according to the stage and resectability of these tumors. Adjuvant CT in resected TET with R0 or R1 resection is not recommended [3,4]. Adjuvant CT is not recommended for resected TETs with R0 or R1 resection [3,4], but rather for unresectable, metastatic, or relapsed TETs. The rarity of TETs explains the lack of randomized phase III trials validating one CT protocol over another. The most commonly used protocols are platinum-based [1,2].

II-1-Induction chemotherapy :

The goal of induction or primary CT in locally advanced TETs is to have a sufficient tumor response to allow for secondary surgical resection or possibly sequential RT [5].

The objective response rate (ORR) and complete response rate (CR) to CT in this case are respectively 50-80% and 30% depending on the series [4,6-8]. The CT protocols used in the literature are essentially based on platinum salts and anthracyclines [9]. In the 1990s, Giaccone et al reported on 5 cases of invasive TET using the PE protocol (Cisplatin 60 mg/m2 ,Etoposide 120 mg/m2×3d)[10]. The ADOC protocol (Doxorubicin 40mg/m2,Cisplatin 50mg/m2, Vincristine 0.6mg/m2 and Cyclophosphamide 700mg/m2) has been retrospectively tested by several teams and proved an ORR ranging from 82% to 100%[6,11,12]. Loehrer et al studied the PAC protocol (Cisplatin 50mg/m2, Doxorubicin 50mg/m2 and Cyclophosphamide 500mg/m2) with 2 to 4 cycles in neoadjuvant followed by RT. The post-CT ORR was 69.6% [13]. Jacot et al reported 6 out of 8 partial responses (PR) with the CAP protocol [14].Yokoi et al reported an ORR of 93% with the CAMP protocol (Cisplatin 20mg/m2d1-d4, Doxorubicin 50mg/m2, Methyl-prednisone1000 mg/d d1-d4 and 500 mg/d , d5-6) as neoadjuvant [15]. Several other neoadjuvant protocols have been studied (Table 1).

Thus, several CT protocols have proven to be effective in neoadjuvant TET. The European Society Of Medical Oncology (ESMO) recommends cisplatin-based CT in this situation, with CAP or PE being the recommended options [16]. The National Comprehensive Cancer Network (NCCN) recommends the CAP protocol in neoadjuvant thymoma in its 2021 version [17].

Table 1: Neoadjuvant chemotherapy protocol and objective response rate :

Authors Year	Chemotherapy	Chemotherapy dose	Type of study	Number of patients	Objective response rate
Macchiarini et al 1991[18]	CEE	Cisplatin 75mg/m2 d1 Epirubicin 100mg/m2 d1 Etoposide 120mg/m2 d1-3	Phase II	7	100%
Shin et al 1998[19][	CAPP	Cyclophosphamide 500 mg/m2/d d1, Doxorubicin 20 mg/m2/d d1-3, Cisplatin 30 mg/m2/d d-3, d1-3 Prednisone 100mg/d*5d	Foresight	12	100%
Loherer et al 2001 [20]	VIP	Etoposide 75 mg/m² x 4d Ifosfamide 1.2 g/m² x 4d Cisplatin 20mg/m2x4d	Phase II	34	32%
Kim et al 2004 [7]	CAPP	Cyclophosphamide 500 mg/m2/d d1, Doxorubicin 20 mg/m2/d d1-3, Cisplatin 30 mg/m2/d d-3, d1-3 Prednisone 100mg/d*5d	Phase II	22	77%
Lemma et al 2008[8]	Carbo-paclitaxel	Carboplatin AUC 6 / 3 Paclitaxel 225 mg/m² / 3	Phase II	46	43%

Kunitoh et al 2009[21]	CODE	S1: Cisplatin 25 mg/m2 d1 Vincristine 1mg/m2 d1, Doxorubicin 40mg/m2 d1, Etoposide 80 mg/m2 d1-3. S2, 4, 6 and 8: Cisplatin 25 mg/m2 d1 Vincristine 1mg/m2 d1, S3,5,7,9: Cisplatin 25 mg/m2 d1 Doxorubicin 40mg/m2 d1, Etoposide 80 mg /m2 on days 1-3.	Phase II	21	62%
Park et al 2013[22]	Cisplatin Docetaxel	Cisplatin 75 mg /m2 Docetaxel 75 mg /m2	Phase II	27	63%

II-2-Palliative or exclusive chemotherapy :

In unresectable metastatic TET, palliative CT may be the only therapeutic modality to be prescribed. The goal of treatment in this case is tumor response and symptom resolution[16,17,23,24]. Multiple lines of palliative CT may also be offered as the sole therapeutic weapon to patients with recurrent or progressive TET [16,17,23,24]. Cisplatin-based CT is recommended in this case [4,5,9]. Merveilleux du Vignaux et al, in a 54 year old series from the Thymic Tumor and Cancer Network (RYTHMIC) who received exclusive CT upfront, noted a lower ORR than induction CT. The ORR was 31% for thymoma and 37% for thymic carcinoma. PAC CT was administered in 67% of cases followed by Carboplatin-

Paclitaxel (20% of cases) and PE (11% of cases) [23]. Loehrer et al, reported an ORR of 50% in a phase II trial of 30 patients with metastatic or recurrent TET with a median survival of 38 months and time to progression of 18.4 months [25].

Taxane-based exclusive CT protocols have proven an ORR ranging from 30 to 60% and are generally proposed for thymic carcinomas [2]. (Table II)

Table II: Exclusive taxane-based chemotherapy and objective response rate

Author Year	Protocol	Type of study	Number of patients	Thymoma/thymic carcinoma	Objective response rate	Therapeutic line
Furugen et al 2011[26]	Carboplatin-Paclitaxel		16	0/16	38%	>1
Lemma et al 2011 [2727]	Carboplatin-Paclitaxel	Phase II	44	21/23	30%	>1
Hirai et al 2015 [2828]	Carboplatin-Paclitaxel	Phase II	39	0/39	36%	No report
Kim et al 2015 [2929]	Cisplatin-Genoxol-PM	Phase II	24	14/28	63%	>1

Giaccone et al conducted a phase II study of the PE protocol in 16 patients with metastatic or recurrent TET. Five complete and four partial responses were obtained with a median duration of response of 3.4 years. The toxicity was acceptable [30].

If relapse occurs, multiple consecutive lines of CT may be used. Readministration of a cytotoxic agent may be considered based on previous efficacy, duration of response, general condition, and cumulative doses for anthracyclines [31].

Several phase II studies have evaluated monoCTs or polyCTs in this situation.

Pemetrexed 500 mg/m2 every 21 days induced 2 partial responses and 2 complete responses in the 23 evaluable patients. The median number of prior therapies was 2. The median time to progression was 45 weeks for thymomas and 5 weeks for thymic carcinomas [32][

Palmieri et al evaluated the combination of capecitabine (650mg/m2*2/d 14d/3S) and gemcitabine (1g/m2 S1-S2) in 30 patients who had received at least one prior line of systemic therapy. They reported a response in 12 patients/30 [33].

II-3-Concurrent chemo-radiotherapy:

Thymic carcinomas are aggressive tumors frequently diagnosed at stage III-IV [34]. The combination of chemo-radiotherapy (CT-RT) would be by extrapolation to other neoplasias an effective therapeutic weapon in this situation. Case studies have been reported in the literature showing the efficacy of concomitant CT-RT in thymic carcinomas [34-36]. This combination allowed secondary surgical resection with complete remission ranging from 15 to 30 months. (Table III). In 2004, Chen et al reported a series of 16 patients with thymic carcinoma (stage III, IVb) treated with concomitant CT- RT. The CT protocol used was either CT with 5 Fluorouracil Cisplatin (Cisplatin 100mg/m2 d1, 5-Fluorouracil1g/m2 d1-d4) or CT with ADOC (Doxorubicin30mg/m2 d1, Cisplatin 50mg/m2 d1, Vincristine 0.6mj/m2 D3, Cyclophosphamide 500 mg/m2 D4). The ORR was 50% with 25% complete response [37].

Table III: Case reports of concomitant chemo-radiotherapy in thymic carcinoma

	Patients	Type	Chemotherapy Protocol	TRO*	surgery	Prognosis
Morio 2002[35]	1	Thymic carcinoma (IVb)	Cisplatin 25mg /m2/S Paclitaxel 80mg/m2/S	61.5%	yes	In RC** at 15 months
Fukuda 2007[34]	1	Thymic carcinoma (IVb)	Paclitaxel:180 mg/m2 Cisplatin:80 mg/m2	PR: 37%.	yes	In RC at 2 years
Kayata 2017[36]	1	Thymic carcinoma (IVb)	Cisplatin:80 mg/m2 Etoposide:100 mg/m2 d1-3	Rp: 65%.	yes	In 30-month CR

ORR: objective response rate, **CR: complete remission

Concomitant CT-RT has been studied in heterogeneous series of TETs involving unresectable advanced thymoma and carcinoma.

In 2008, Wright et al. reported a series of 10 patients with stage III-IVA TET. These patients underwent concomitant CT-RT with 2 cycles of EP followed by surgery. Eight patients had R0 and two R1 resections. Tumor necrosis > 90% was noted in 4 cases. Seven patients received 2 additional cycles of adjuvant CT. The overall survival at 5 years was 69% [38].The promising results of this study led Korst et al to launch a phase II trial studying the histological response after concomitant CT-RT followed by surgery. This trial included 21 patients. 17 had R0 resection. There was no complete histological response. However, 24% of TETs had less than 10% viable cells [39].

Recently, a Chinese phase trial studied concomitant CT-RT with EP (Etoposide 75 mg/m2, Cisplatin 25 mg/m2 d1-3), 2 cycles concurrent with RT, 2 cycles after RT. This trial included 56 patients followed for unresectable advanced TET. 85.7% of patients had stage IV TET. The ORR was 85.7%. With a median follow-up of 46 months, the PFS and OS at 5 years were respectively 29.5% and 56.2% with acceptable toxicity. RT was intensity modulated radiation [40].

III. Targeted therapies:

During the last decade, several targeted therapies approved in other solid tumors have been studied in previously treated TETs [24]. These targeted therapies have shown variable ORR in [2nd] line therapy.

c-KIT is often overexpressed in thymic carcinomas (79-88%) but an activating mutation is found in less than 10% of cases [24,41,42]. Phase II trials evaluating the efficacy of Imatinib in TETs were disappointing [43,44].

Anti-angiogenic drugs have proven to be effective in second-line thymic carcinoma [45,46]. The Italian Association of Medical Oncology (AIOM) and ESMO have proposed Sunitinib as a second-line option for thymic carcinoma [16,47].

Everolimus (an mTOR inhibitor) has shown promising results in a Phase II trial. Indeed, with a median follow-up of 25.7 months, the median progression-free survival and overall survival were 10.1 months (16.6 months for thymoma and 5.6 months for thymic carcinoma) and 25.7 months (not reached for thymoma and 14.7 months for thymic carcinoma) respectively [48]. The American NCCN guidelines propose Everolimus as a second-line treatment option and the European guidelines propose it as an option for refractory TETs [16,17].

Table IV summarizes the phase II trials showing the efficacy of antiangiogenic drugs and mTOR inhibitor in pretreated TET.

Table IV: Phase II trials validating targeted therapies in thymic epithelial tumors

Author Year	Targeted therapy	Number of patients	Reverse	Evaluation
Bedano et al 2008 [4949]	Erlotinib +Bevacizumab	18		DM: 50% of cases
Thomas et al 2015 [4545]	Sunitinib	23 TC	17 months	DM 65%. PR: 26%. PM: 9%.
		16 T	17 months	DM 75%. PR: 6%. PM: 19%.
Zucali et al 2018 [4848]	Everolimus	32 T 19 TC	25.7 months	RC: 1 TC RP: 3T, 2 CT SM: 38, (27T, 11CT) MCT:88%.
Sato et al 2020 [4646]	Levatinib	42 TC	15.5 months	Stability: 57%. PR: 38%.

T: Thymoma, TC: Thymic carcinoma, SM: stable disease, PR: partial response, PM: disease progression, TCM: disease control rate

Somatostatin analogues have also been studied in thymoma with a positive octreotide scan [50]. The combination of Octreotide and Prednisone further improves the ORR [51-54]. (Table V). The trials with octreotide included patients previously treated with systemic therapy. In the study by Kirzinger et al, patients had unresectable stage III disease of primary discovery or relapse (1 patient had RT and 3 patients had previously received CT)

Table V: Objective response rates to octreotide plus or minus prednisone

Author Year	Type of study	Number of patients	Study protocol	TRO	SG, SGM, TTPM
Palmieri et al 2002[51][	Phase II	16	Octreotide s/c:0.5 mg*3/ day +PDN:0.6 mg/kg/day	37%	MGS: 15 months TTPM: 14 months
Loehrer et al 2004[5252]	Phase II	38	Octreotide/c:0.5 mg*3/ day *02 months associated beyond if no answer atPDN :0.6 mg/kg/day	31.6%	SG to: 1 year 87 2 years: 76%.
Longo et al 2012[54]	Retrospective	12	Octreotide LAR: 20mg IM/every 15 days	25%	TTPM: 8 months
Kirzinger et al 2012[53]	Phase II	17	OctreotideLAR: 30 mg IM/ every 15 days +PDN: 0.6 mg/kg/day	88%	

PDN: prednisone, ORR: objective response rate, OS: overall survival, MOS: median overall survival, TTPM: median time to progression

IV- Immunotherapy:

The rationale for the use of PD1/ PD-L1 checkpoint inhibitors (CPIs) is based on its high expression in TETs. PDL1 is expressed in 23-92% of thymomas and 36-100% of thymic carcinomas [55,56]. A few phase II trials have investigated the use of CPIs in refractory TETs. The main evidence for the use of pembrolizumab comes from a US study. Giaccone et al, showed an ORR of 22.5% to pembrolizumab in a population of 41 patients followed for relapsed thymic carcinoma. The median duration of response was 22.4 months. Disease stability was found in 53% of cases. The overall survival at 1 year was 71%. Six patients (15% of cases) presented severe autoimmune disorders, including 2 myocarditis

[57]. A similar study was conducted in Chorea. Cho et al. described an ORR of 19.2% in thymic carcinomas and 28.6% in thymomas. The disease was stable in thymoma and thymic carcinoma in 72% and 54% of cases respectively. The median progression-free survival was 6.1 months in both groups. A serious autoimmune adverse event was found in 71% of thymomas and 15% of carcinomas [58]. These two studies prove the activity of immunotherapy in TETs at the cost of a sometimes serious toxicity despite a prior assessment of autoimmunity. Thus, the American and Italian learned societies propose pembrolizumab as a second-line systemic treatment for thymic carcinomas [17, 47].

V- Conclusion:

Systemic treatment in TETs is discussed whenever the tumor is locally advanced, metastatic or in relapse. Today, we have several lines of treatment: CT, targeted therapy, immunotherapy. However, cisplatin-based CT remains the standard treatment to be proposed in the first line. The other systemic therapeutic weapons should be proposed in the second line.

References:

1. Kelly RJ, Petrini I, Rajan A, Wang Y, Giaccone G. Thymic Malignancies: From Clinical Management to Targeted Therapies. J Clin Oncol. 2011 Dec 20;29(36):4820-7.

2. Berghmans T, Durieux V, Holbrechts S, Jungels C, Lafitte J-J, Meert A-P, et al. Systemic treatments for thymoma and thymic carcinoma: A systematic review. Lung Cancer Amst Neth. Dec 2018;126:25-31.

3. Scorsetti M, Leo F, Trama A, D'Angelillo R, Serpico D, Macerelli M, et al. Thymoma and thymic carcinomas. Crit Rev Oncol Hematol. march 2016;99:332-50.

4. Valente M, Schinzari G, Ricciotti A, Barone C. Role of chemotherapy in malignant thymoma. Ann Ital Chir. Oct 2007;78(5):377-80.

5. Rajan A, Giaccone G. Chemotherapy for thymic tumors: induction, consolidation, palliation. Thorac Surg Clin. Feb 2011;21(1):107-14, viii.

6. Berruti A, Borasio P, Gerbino A, Gorzegno G, Moschini T, Tampellini M, et al. Primary chemotherapy with adriamycin, cisplatin, vincristine and cyclophosphamide in locally advanced thymomas: a single institution experience. Br J Cancer. Nov 1999;81(5):841-5.

7. Kim ES, Putnam JB, Komaki R, Walsh GL, Ro JY, Shin HJ, et al. Phase II study of a multidisciplinary approach with induction chemotherapy, followed by surgical resection, radiation therapy, and consolidation chemotherapy for unresectable malignant thymomas: final report. Lung Cancer Amst Neth. June 2004;44(3):369-79.

8. Lemma GL, Lee J-W, Aisner SC, Langer CJ, Tester WJ, Johnson DH, et al. Phase II study of carboplatin and paclitaxel in advanced thymoma and thymic carcinoma. J Clin Oncol Off J Am Soc Clin Oncol. May 20, 2011;29(15):2060-5.

9. Okuma Y, Saito M, Hosomi Y, Sakuyama T, Okamura T. Key components of chemotherapy for thymic malignancies: a systematic review and pooled analysis for anthracycline-, carboplatin- or cisplatin-based chemotherapy. J Cancer Res Clin Oncol. Feb 2015;141(2):323-31.

10. Giaccone G, Musella R, Bertetto O, Donadio M, Calciati A. Cisplatin-containing chemotherapy in the treatment of invasive thymoma: report of five cases. Cancer Treat Rep. June 1985;69(6):695-7.

11. Fornasiero A, Daniele O, Ghiotto C, Piazza M, Fiore-Donati L, Calabró F, et al. Chemotherapy for invasive thymoma. A 13-year experience. Cancer. July 1, 1991;68(1):30-3.

12. Rea F, Sartori F, Loy M, Calabrò F, Fornasiero A, Daniele O, et al. Chemotherapy and operation for invasive thymoma. J Thorac Cardiovasc Surg. Sept 1993;106(3):543-9.

13. Loehrer PJ, Chen M, Kim K, Aisner SC, Einhorn LH, Livingston R, et al. Cisplatin, doxorubicin, and cyclophosphamide plus thoracic radiation therapy for limited-stage unresectable thymoma: an intergroup trial. J Clin Oncol. 1997 Sep 1;15(9):3093-9.

14. Jacot W, Quantin X, Valette S, Khial F, Pujol JL. Multimodality Treatment Program in Invasive Thymic Epithelial Tumor. Am J Clin Oncol. Feb 2005;28(1):5-7.

15. Yokoi K, Matsuguma H, Nakahara R, Kondo T, Kamiyama Y, Mori K, et al. Multidisciplinary treatment for advanced invasive thymoma with cisplatin, doxorubicin, and methylprednisolone. J Thorac Oncol Off Publ Int Assoc Study Lung Cancer. Jan 2007;2(1):73-8.

16. Girard N, Ruffini E, Marx A, Faivre-Finn C, Peters S. Thymic epithelial tumours: ESMO Clinical Practice Guidelines for diagnosis, treatment and follow-up. Ann Oncol. Sep 2015;26:v40-55.

17. thymic.pdf [Internet]. [cited 9 Jul 2021]. Available from: https://www.nccn.org/professionals/physician_gls/pdf/thymic.pdf

18. Macchiarini P, Chella A, Ducci F, Rossi B, Testi C, Bevilacqua G, et al. Neoadjuvant chemotherapy, surgery, and postoperative radiation therapy for invasive thymoma. Cancer. August 15, 1991;68(4):706-13.

19. Shin DM. A Multidisciplinary Approach to Therapy for Unresectable Malignant Thymoma. Ann Intern Med. 1998 Jul 15;129(2):100.

20. Loehrer PJ, Jiroutek M, Aisner S, Aisner J, Green M, Thomas CR, et al. Combined etoposide, ifosfamide, and cisplatin in the treatment of patients with advanced thymoma and thymic carcinoma: an intergroup trial. Cancer. June 1, 2001;91(11):2010-5.

21. Kunitoh H, Tamura T, Shibata T, Takeda K, Katakami N, Nakagawa K, et al. A phase II trial of dose-dense chemotherapy, followed by surgical resection and/or thoracic radiotherapy, in locally advanced thymoma: report of a Japan Clinical Oncology Group trial (JCOG 9606). Br J Cancer. June 29, 2010;103(1):6-11.

22. Park S, Ahn M, Ahn JS, Sun J-M, Shim YM, Kim J, et al. A prospective phase II trial of induction chemotherapy with docetaxel/cisplatin for Masaoka stage III/IV thymic epithelial tumors. J Thorac Oncol Off Publ Int Assoc Study Lung Cancer. jul 2013;8(7):959-66.

23. Merveilleux du Vignaux C, Dansin E, Mhanna L, Greillier L, Pichon E, Kerjouan M, et al. Systemic Therapy in Advanced Thymic Epithelial Tumors: Insights from the RYTHMIC Prospective Cohort. J Thorac Oncol. nov 2018;13(11):1762-70.

24. Drevet G, Collaud S, Tronc F, Girard N, Maury J-M. Optimal management of thymic malignancies: current perspectives. Cancer Manag Res. 2019;11:6803-14.

25. Loehrer PJ, Kim K, Aisner SC, Livingston R, Einhorn LH, Johnson D, et al. Cisplatin plus doxorubicin plus cyclophosphamide in metastatic or recurrent thymoma: final results of an intergroup trial. The Eastern Cooperative Oncology Group, Southwest Oncology Group, and Southeastern Cancer Study Group. J Clin Oncol Off J Am Soc Clin Oncol. June 1994;12(6):1164-8.

26. Furugen M, Sekine I, Tsuta K, Horinouchi H, Nokihara H, Yamamoto N, et al. Combination Chemotherapy with Carboplatin and Paclitaxel for Advanced Thymic Cancer. Jpn J Clin Oncol. 2011 Aug 1;41(8):1013-6.

27. Lemma GL, Loehrer PJ, Lee JW, Langer CJ, Tester WJ, Johnson DH. A phase II study of carboplatin plus paclitaxel in advanced thymoma or thymic carcinoma: E1C99. J Clin Oncol. May 20, 2008;26(15_suppl):8018-8018.

28. Hirai F, Yamanaka T, Taguchi K, Daga H, Ono A, Tanaka K, et al. A multicenter phase II study of carboplatin and paclitaxel for advanced thymic carcinoma: WJOG4207L. Ann Oncol Off J Eur Soc Med Oncol. Feb 2015;26(2):363-8.

29. Kim HS, Lee JY, Lim SH, Sun J-M, Lee SH, Ahn JS, et al. A Prospective Phase II Study of Cisplatin and Cremophor EL-Free Paclitaxel (Genexol-PM) in Patients with Unresectable Thymic Epithelial Tumors. J Thorac Oncol Off Publ Int Assoc Study Lung Cancer. dec 2015;10(12):1800-6.

30. Giaccone G, Ardizzoni A, Kirkpatrick A, Clerico M, Sahmoud T, van Zandwijk N. Cisplatin and etoposide combination chemotherapy for locally advanced or metastatic thymoma. A phase II study of the European Organization for Research and Treatment of Cancer Lung Cancer Cooperative Group. J Clin Oncol Off J Am Soc Clin Oncol. March 1996;14(3):814-20.

31. Lara PN, Bonomi PD, Faber LP. Retreatment of recurrent invasive thymoma with platinum, doxorubicin, and cyclophosphamide. Chest. Oct 1996;110(4):1115-7.

32. Loehrer PJ, Yiannoutsos CT, Dropcho S, Burns M, Helft P, Chiorean EG, et al. A phase II trial of pemetrexed in patients with recurrent thymoma or thymic carcinoma. J Clin Oncol. 2006 Jun 20;24(18_suppl):7079-7079.

33. Palmieri G, Buonerba C, Ottaviano M, Federico P, Calabrese F, Von Arx C, et al. Capecitabine plus gemcitabine in thymic epithelial tumors: final analysis of a Phase II trial. Future Oncol Lond Engl. Nov 2014;10(14):2141-7.

34. Fukuda M, Obase Y, Miyashita N, Kobashi Y, Mohri K, Ueno S, et al. Paclitaxel and Cisplatin with Concurrent Radiotherapy followed by Surgery in Locally Advanced Thymic Carcinoma. ANTICANCER Res. 2007;4.

35. Morio A, Nakahara K, Ohse Y, Tahara M, Goto T, Yakumaru K, et al. Efficacy of induction chemoradiotherapy in thymic cancer: report of a successful case and review of the literature. Int J Clin Oncol. June 1, 2002;7(3):201-4.

36. Kayata H, Isaka M, Ohde Y, Takahashi T, Harada H. Complete Resection of Masaoka Stage IVb Thymic Carcinoma After Chemoradiotherapy. Ann Thorac Surg. jan 2017;103(1):e5-7.

37. Chen Y-Y, Huang C-H, Tang Y, Eng H-L. Concurrent Chemoradiotherapy for Unresectable Thymic Carcinoma. 2004;27(7):8.

38. Wright CD, Choi NC, Wain JC, Mathisen DJ, Lynch TJ, Fidias P. Induction Chemoradiotherapy Followed by Resection for Locally Advanced Masaoka Stage III and IVA Thymic Tumors. Ann Thorac Surg. Feb 2008;85(2):385-9.

39. Korst RJ, Bezjak A, Blackmon S, Choi N, Fidias P, Liu G, et al. Neoadjuvant chemoradiotherapy for locally advanced thymic tumors: A phase II, multi-institutional clinical trial. J Thorac Cardiovasc Surg. jan 2014;147(1):36-46.e1.

40. Fan X-W, Yang Y, Wang H-B, Xu Y, Kang M, Xie L-Y, et al. Intensity Modulated Radiation Therapy Plus Etoposide/Cisplatin for Patients With Limited Advanced Unresectable Thymic Epithelial Tumors: A Prospective Phase 2 Study. Int J Radiat Oncol. May 2020;107(1):98-105.

41. Tateo V, Manuzzi L, Parisi C, De Giglio A, Campana D, Pantaleo MA, et al. An Overview on Molecular Characterization of Thymic Tumors: Old and New Targets for Clinical Advances. Pharmaceuticals. Apr 1, 2021;14(4):316.

42. Girard N, Shen R, Guo T, Zakowski MF, Heguy A, Riely GJ, et al. Comprehensive genomic analysis reveals clinically relevant molecular distinctions between thymic carcinomas and thymomas. Clin Cancer Res Off J Am Assoc Cancer Res. 2009 Nov 15;15(22):6790-9.

43. Palmieri G, Marino M, Buonerba C, Federico P, Conti S, Milella M, et al. Imatinib mesylate in thymic epithelial malignancies. Cancer Chemother Pharmacol. 1 Feb 2012;69(2):309-15.

44. Giaccone G, Rajan A, Ruijter R, Smit E, van Groeningen C, Hogendoorn PCW. Imatinib mesylate in patients with WHO B3 thymomas and thymic

carcinomas. J Thorac Oncol Off Publ Int Assoc Study Lung Cancer. Oct 2009;4(10):1270-3.

45. Thomas A, Rajan A, Berman A, Tomita Y, Brzezniak C, Lee M-J, et al. Sunitinib in patients with chemotherapy-refractory thymoma and thymic carcinoma: an open-label phase 2 trial. Lancet Oncol. Feb 2015;16(2):177-86.

46. Sato J, Satouchi M, Itoh S, Okuma Y, Niho S, Mizugaki H, et al. Lenvatinib in patients with advanced or metastatic thymic carcinoma (REMORA): a multicentre, phase 2 trial. Lancet Oncol. June 2020;21(6):843-50.

47. Conforti F, Marino M, Vitolo V, Spaggiari L, Mantegazza R, Zucali P, et al. Clinical management of patients with thymic epithelial tumors: the recommendations endorsed by the Italian Association of Medical Oncology (AIOM). ESMO Open. June 8, 2021;6(4):100188.

48. Zucali PA, De Pas T, Palmieri G, Favaretto A, Chella A, Tiseo M, et al. Phase II Study of Everolimus in Patients With Thymoma and Thymic Carcinoma Previously Treated With Cisplatin-Based Chemotherapy. J Clin Oncol Off J Am Soc Clin Oncol. 1 Feb 2018;36(4):342-9.

49. Bedano PM, Perkins S, Burns M, Kessler K, Nelson R, Schneider BP, et al. A phase II trial of erlotinib plus bevacizumab in patients with recurrent thymoma or thymic carcinoma. J Clin Oncol. May 20, 2008;26(15_suppl):19087-19087.

50. Palmieri G, Montella L, Lastoria S. [Thymoma and somatostatin analogs. Biology, diagnosis and clinical practice]. Minerva Endocrinol. Sept 2001;26(3):193-5.

51. Palmieri G, Montella L, Martignetti A, Muto P, Vizio DD, Chiara AD, et al. Somatostatin analogs and prednisone in advanced refractory thymic tumors. Cancer. 2002;94(5):1414-20.

52. Loehrer PJ, Wang W, Johnson DH, Aisner SC, Ettinger DS, Eastern Cooperative Oncology Group Phase II Trial. Octreotide alone or with prednisone in patients with advanced thymoma and thymic carcinoma: an Eastern Cooperative Oncology Group Phase II Trial. J Clin Oncol Off J Am Soc Clin Oncol. 15 Jan 2004;22(2):293-9.

53. Kirzinger L, Boy S, Marienhagen J, Schuierer G, Neu R, Ried M, et al. Octreotide LAR and Prednisone as Neoadjuvant Treatment in Patients with

Primary or Locally Recurrent Unresectable Thymic Tumors: A Phase II Study. PLOS ONE. 16 Dec 2016;11(12):e0168215.

54. Longo F, De Filippis L, Zivi A, Vitolo D, Del Signore E, Gori B, et al. Efficacy and tolerability of long-acting octreotide in the treatment of thymic tumors: results of a pilot trial. Am J Clin Oncol. Apr 2012;35(2):105-9.

55. Zhao C, Rajan A. Immune checkpoint inhibitors for treatment of thymic epithelial tumors: how to maximize benefit and optimize risk? Mediastinum Hong Kong China. Sep 2019;3:35.

56. Jakopovic M, Bitar L, Seiwerth F, Marusic A, Krpina K, Samarzija M. Immunotherapy for thymoma. J Thorac Dis. Dec 2020;12(12):7635-41.

57. Giaccone G, Kim C, Thompson J, McGuire C, Kallakury B, Chahine JJ, et al. Pembrolizumab in patients with thymic carcinoma: a single-arm, single-centre, phase 2 study. Lancet Oncol. march 2018;19(3):347-55.

58. Cho J, Kim HS, Ku BM, Choi Y-L, Cristescu R, Han J, et al. Pembrolizumab for Patients With Refractory or Relapsed Thymic Epithelial Tumor: An Open-Label Phase II Trial. J Clin Oncol Off J Am Soc Clin Oncol. August 20, 2019;37(24):2162-70.

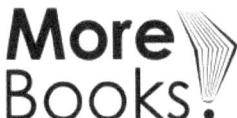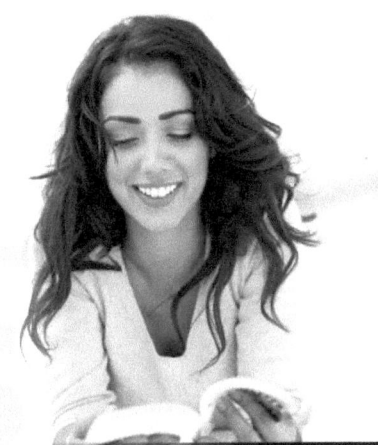

I want morebooks!

Buy your books fast and straightforward online - at one of world's fastest growing online book stores! Environmentally sound due to Print-on-Demand technologies.

Buy your books online at
www.morebooks.shop

Kaufen Sie Ihre Bücher schnell und unkompliziert online – auf einer der am schnellsten wachsenden Buchhandelsplattformen weltweit! Dank Print-On-Demand umwelt- und ressourcenschonend produziert.

Bücher schneller online kaufen
www.morebooks.shop

 info@omniscriptum.com
www.omniscriptum.com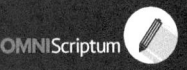

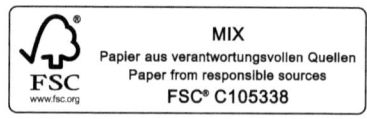

Printed by Books on Demand GmbH, Norderstedt / Germany